DEVELOPING MENTAL TOUGHNESS

DEVELOPING MENTAL TOUGHNESS

Gold Medal Strategies for Transforming Your Business Performance

Graham Jones & Adrian Moorhouse MBE

Viva Books

New Delhi | Mumbai | Chennai | Kolkata | Bengaluru | Hyderabad | Kochi | Guwahati

First Indian Edition 2010

VIVA BOOKS PRIVATE LIMITED

- 4737/23 Ansari Road, Daryaganj, New Delhi 110 002
  E-mail: vivadelhi@vivagroupindia.net, Tel. 42242200
- 76, Service Industries, Shirvane, Sector 1, Nerul, Navi Mumbai 400 706
  E-mail: vivamumbai@vivagroupindia.net, Tel. 27721273, 27721274
- Jamals Fazal Chambers, 26 Greams Road, Chennai 600 006
  E-mail: vivachennai@vivagroupindia.net, Tel. 28290304, 28294241
- B-103, Jindal Towers, 21/1A/3 Darga Road, Kolkata 700 017
  E-mail: vivakolkata@vivagroupindia.net, Tel. 22836381, 22816713
- 7, Sovereign Park Apartments, 56-58, K. R. Road, Basavanagudi, Bengaluru 560 004
  E-mail: vivabangalore@vivagroupindia.net, Tel. 26607409, 26607410
- 101-102 Mughal Marc Apartments, 3-4-637 to 641, Narayanguda, Hyderabad 500 029
  E-mail: vivahyderabad@vivagroupindia.net, Tel. 27564481, 27564482
- Beevi Towers, First Floor, SRM Road, Kaloor, Kochi 682 018, Kerala
  E-mail: vivakochi@vivagroupindia.net, Tel: 0484-2403055, 2403056
- 232, GNB Road, Beside UCO Bank, Silpukhuri, Guwahati 781 003
  E-mail: vivaguwahati@vivagroupindia.net, Tel: 0361-2666386

www.vivagroupindia.com

Published by arrangement with
How to Books
Spring Hill House, Spring Hill Road
Begbroke, Oxford OX5 1RX,
United Kingdom

NOTE: The material contained in this book is set out in good faith for general guidance and no liability can be accepted for loss or expense incurred as a result of relying in particular circumstances on statements made in the book. The laws and regulations are complex and liable to change, and readers should check the current position with the relevant authorited before making personal arrangements.

ISBN : 978-81-309-1464-0

Published by Vinod Vasishtha for Viva Books Private Limited, 4737/23, Ansari Road, New Delhi-110 002. Printed and bound by Swan Press, New Delhi.

M0000

Contents

List of illustrations

About the Authors

Professor Graham Jones is a founding Director of Lane4 Management Group Ltd. He was formerly a Reader in Sport Psychology at Loughborough University for 11 years before becoming Professor of Elite Performance Psychology at the University of Wales, Bangor. He has over 100 publications in the area of high level performance, including books on stress and performance and the psychology of elite performance and a recent article in *Harvard Business Review*. He is also a former Editor of the international journal, *The Sport Psychologist*. Graham is a Chartered Psychologist with the British Psychological Society and a Registered Sport Psychologist with the British Olympic Association. His applied work includes consulting with numerous elite performers, including World Champions and Olympic medal winners, professional golfers on the European Tour, the 1996 GB Olympic team, the Wales rugby union team, the British Bobsleigh Association, the Great Britain hockey team and the Royal Marines. He has also worked with individual world-ranked performers from a variety of sports, including squash, swimming, football, judo, ice skating, track and field athletics, rugby league, motor racing, cricket, snooker and trampolining. Graham's experience of working with business executives spans over ten years, and includes working closely with company boards as well as on large scale initiatives around culture change, mergers and global roll-outs of people development programmes. Some of the organisations he has worked with include Ericsson, Fujitsu, Coca-Cola Enterprises, The Coca Cola Company, Safeway, Lloyds TSB, Bourne Leisure, JP Morgan, HSBC, Deutsche Bank, Roche Pharmaceuticals, Daimler Chrysler, CRH, Woolworths, Capita Symonds, 3M, the UK Atomic Energy Authority, Sainsburys, easyJet, Accenture, Invesco, Dyson, St. Mary's Hospital, Paddington, Merrill Lynch, UBS, National Grid, Honda, Linklaters and Goldman Sachs.

Adrian Moorhouse MBE retired in 1992 from a career unparalleled in British swimming, with twelve years at international level highlighted by an Olympic gold medal at the Seoul Olympic Games and sustaining his World Number One ranking for 6 years. Adrian was also the European

Champion 4 consecutive times and Commonwealth Games Gold Medallist in three Games. He broke the World Record over 5 times and held it for over 5 years. In 1987, he was awarded an MBE for his services to swimming. A former Radio 4 children's show presenter, his work in the field of sport is still ongoing as a swimming commentator for the BBC and as a patron of SPARKS charity. Adrian is now the Managing Director and co-founder of Lane4 Management Group, a successful international performance development consultancy. Adrian's role at Lane4 centres around shaping Lane4 as a business and driving company growth whilst ensuring the maintenance of strong client relationships and the delivery of high quality products. Some of the organisations that Adrian has worked with include Honda, Sainsbury's, SJ Berwin, Deutsche Bank, Microsoft MSN, Accenture, DSM, Exxon Mobil, Bourne Leisure, Curry's, Budget, Roche Pharmaceuticals, Lloyds TSB, Safeway, Bausch & Lomb and Manchester Airport PLC.

Acknowledgements

We would like to give a special thanks to Sam Walker for her support and drive in ensuring that this book got finished.

We are also very grateful to the following people for their help and support, provided in a variety of different ways, in producing this book: Dr Tara Jones, Martin Rogan, Clare Garbett, Matt Rogan, Kellie Johnston, Professor Sheldon Hanton, Dr Declan Connaughton and Penny Gray.

To Tara and Liz. Thank you for your love, support and tolerance.

1 Introduction

Sport is a powerful metaphor for business. Fierce competition, winning by sometimes the smallest margins, achieving goals and targets, establishing long-term and short-term strategies and tactics, hard work, perseverance, determination, teamwork, dealing with success and recovering from failure and setbacks are all key elements of both worlds. Underpinning success in sport and business is the ability to continually move performance to higher levels – what you achieve this year is never going to be good enough next year. Goals and standards move onwards and upwards, resulting in an incessant demand to find new means and methods to ensure the delivery of performance curves that at times can seem tantalisingly, and at other times impossibly, out of reach. These constitute the essential ingredients of pressure, and achieving sustainable high performance under pressure requires you to be mentally tough.

Adrian and I have some valuable and fascinating insights into mental toughness based on our combined knowledge and experience of studying and consulting with some of the world's best performers, in my case and, in Adrian's case, actually being one of them! We have wrestled with how best to communicate what is essentially an explicit understanding of the psychology of high achievers based on researching and supporting them, combined with an implicit awareness of how to achieve World Number One status and sustain it over six consecutive years.

Our conclusion is that Adrian and I should present these perspectives separately. We each have our own stories to tell so the remainder of the book is written in the context of our own personal and different perspectives. This is largely in the form of:

- my identification, explanation and guidance on how to develop and enhance the essential elements of mental toughness;
- with Adrian's inputs highlighting and bringing alive the key messages and principles involved.

The remainder of this introduction tells the stories of how we came to be so heavily involved in elite sport and how our respective consulting and high achiever worlds collided to form such a powerful perspective on how to deliver sustainable high performance. It then goes on to outline the content and layout of the book and how to get the most from it.

Adrian's story

As a child of 12, it was my biggest dream ever since seeing David Wilkie win the 200 metres breaststroke in 1976 to win a Gold Medal at the Olympic Games. I spent the next eight years training and competing at various levels from county to district to national, achieving quite rapid success.

Olympic Gold Medallist

I first represented the Great Britain senior team in 1980 at the age of 15, and carried on making such rapid progress that at the start of the 1984 Olympic year I was already European Champion and Commonwealth Games Gold Medal winner. I was ranked as one of the favourites going into the Los Angeles Olympics in July. From the start of that year I began to feel weighed down by my own expectations; this was my chance to fulfil my dream and also other people's expectations. I remember reading in the newspaper how I was going to carry on the British tradition of Olympic Gold Medal breaststroke winners – 'Wilkie '76, Goodhew '80, Moorhouse '84?'

Every race I swam, and indeed every training session I did, became so very important. In fact I over-magnified the importance of every session and every race. Indeed, I came to think that any perceived weakness in the last four months would lead to my ultimate failure. It reached such an extent that in April I was sleeping very fitfully for a maximum of four or five hours at a time. I didn't know how to cope with the amount of pressure I placed on myself. Even at the Olympics in Los Angeles, having qualified for the final, I remember sitting in the 'ready room' half an hour before the race feeling that there was no way I could win. I just didn't have the tools to cope with the mental pressure. Needless to say, I didn't win and came an uninspiring fourth. To me that was a failure; I got the same medal as the person who came last – nothing!

The press were equally scathing afterwards, labelling me a failure and suggesting I retire (at the age of 20). My self-belief hit an all-time low and for the next four months my swimming results just got worse. My motivation to train was almost non-existent. I just went because I knew where the swimming pool was and because my friends were there.

One of the keys to rebuilding my self-belief was appreciating some of my past successes and it took my coach's help to work through that with me, to make me appreciate that I had achieved quite a lot. The other thing that helped me was rebuilding some short-term goals to include things I thought I could achieve rather than aiming for the big Olympic Gold Medal again; it was just too daunting. It took me a couple of years and more successes to start to believe that the Gold Medal was within my control again. I was developing a lot of the skills associated with mental toughness.

By 1986 I had achieved the World Number One position and held this through to 1988, the next Olympics in Seoul. I had not changed much of my physical training, but had spent a lot of time developing my mental skills and capabilities. Walking into the final of the 100 metres breaststroke, I believed I was going to win and knew how to handle the pressure, either self-imposed or press-related! It was not a foregone conclusion, but I did actually win that race. One significant moment to test my belief was at the halfway turn where I was in sixth place out of eight. I drew on past experience and belief in my capabilities for a strong last 25 metres and banished negative thoughts from my head. I went on to win the race by just one hundredth of a second.

I am sure that developing the key skills around belief, motivation, focus and the ability to handle pressure was the key factor. In other words, I had become mentally tough.

My swimming career continued through to the next Olympics in 1992, and I spent most of those four years with a goal of breaking the World Record and reducing it to an unattainable (for other people!) time. I had shifted my main goal and this motivated me for those years. I stayed at the top of the world rankings until 1991 and broke the World Record three times. By the time of the 1992 Olympic year, however, I had slipped to second in the world and started to feel the youngsters quite literally snapping at my heels! I finished eighth in that Olympic final and retired soon afterwards as I felt that my years at the top had come to an end, and I was fulfilled with my career and achievements.

My first job after retiring was working with the English Amateur Swimming Association to create a Junior Talent Development Programme. I also started work with the British Olympic Association to create a Lifestyle Planning Programme for Olympic athletes. For a while I struggled to work out where a future career might lie, but a lot of it came down to just having confidence and belief in myself and staying focused on the job in hand. In reality, I was managing this transition by using all the elements of mental toughness I had learned.

Managing Director

During these first few years after retiring, I had also carried on delivering the odd 'motivational' speech to various businesses. Whilst being financially lucrative, retelling my story soon became empty for me. I found myself wondering what the long-term value might be to those listening, realising that actually it was simply a form of entertainment. I soon realised that I needed a career, and being an entertainer wasn't it.

This coincided with meeting Graham in a bathroom in Florida. We were both working for the British Olympic Association on the preparation camp for the Atlanta Olympics, and our rudimentary accommodation at Florida State University meant that we had to share a bathroom! Over a beer later on, we discussed the key factors that underpin success in sport and their transferability into business. I expressed feeling unsure of the learning I could get across from a stage, and Graham talked passionately about the work he had been doing with business managers in much the same way as he would with a group of elite athletes – over a sustained period and including both group and one-to-one sessions. I realised almost immediately that this was the business opportunity and career that I had been looking for.

In 1995 we started Lane4 with the express aim of bringing some of those tools and skills that I had found so useful to business people around the world. Over the past 12 years we have been working together developing into a more fully-fledged performance consultancy. As I have grown into my new career and role as the Managing Director, I have discovered that there are many similar challenges in running a growing business, for example staying focused on the strategy and goals, and coping with the pressure of the vagaries of the market or competitive environment, as well as my own belief in our proposition and my ability as the leader. Not surprisingly, of all my 'old' skills, it isn't being able to swim fast that has had most impact on my capabilities as a business leader, but my mental toughness.

Graham's story

Have you ever been in a situation in which you knew that if you could summon up the courage to take on a really big challenge it could change your life? It happened to me a number of years ago when I was firmly and comfortably ensconced within the world of academia. I was busy doing what academics do to advance their careers – engrossing myself in research and writing up the findings for publication in peer-reviewed scientific journals. My particular interest in the psychology of elite performance was fuelled by a passion to explore what makes the world's best sport performers tick and, in particular, how they deal with the extraordinary pressure they find themselves surrounded by. This interest in elite performance didn't stop at examining and understanding the key psychological principles of success. I was also working in the real world, consulting with elite performers from a wide variety of sports who were searching for the psychological edge they believed would catapult, or at the very least nudge, them ahead of their rivals.

Applying the psychology of elite performance to business

Then came the day that triggered a chain of events that persuaded me to consider, question and eventually leave behind my comfortable existence. I and my colleague, Dr Austin Swain[1], were approached by David, a senior executive in a large global company, who was seeking to apply the elite sport metaphor to help his already successful senior management team step up to an even higher performance level. This presented an intriguing challenge at one level, because I had often pondered how well the principles of elite sport performance would transfer to other performance arenas.

At another level I was fearful that our relative naivety and lack of experience of the business world would present too much of an obstacle to us in delivering real value to what I anticipated would be a busy group of people with better things to do with their time. And what could Austin and I add to what wasn't already available within their own organisation? This was a huge, well-respected company with a highly-developed human resource department that surely must have ample internal knowledge and experience of the essential principles of performance

[1] Dr Swain is now a fellow Director at Lane4 and was psychologist to the England rugby union team from 1994 to 1997.

management! David, on the other hand, was convinced that we could help, citing the large number of similarities between performance in business and sport as the foundation of his confidence.

I will always be grateful to David and his team for their interest and encouragement as we ventured nervously into what for us was uncharted territory. They too believed that there was something valuable in what we had to say and offer, and as I got to grips with 'P'n Ls', 'PDRs', 'PDPs', '360 feedback' and other terminology that seemed baffling at the time, so my confidence grew and I felt that we were making an impact. In fact the work with David's team had very positive results and it did prove to be that life-changing experience for me. Here was another type of environment hungry for the basics of performance psychology and it was a very responsive environment ready to experiment with many of the key principles of elite sport performance. The crucial factor and learning for me was that the principles applied extremely well to the business environment.

There was actually a second part to this life-changing event, although I didn't recognise it as such at the time. During my work with the British Olympic Association in helping to prepare the Great Britain team for the 1996 Olympics, I had met former Olympic swimming Gold Medallist, Adrian Moorhouse. As well as his Olympic Gold Medal success, Adrian had been ranked as World Number One for six consecutive years before his retirement in 1992. He had also been applying his vast experience and knowledge of performing at the highest level in sport to business, but Adrian was conscious that he was telling a story of how he succeeded without ever truly understanding the key principles that underpinned it.

We talked at length about how his thoughts, attitudes and behaviours fitted around things like motivation, belief, goal setting, focus and handling pressure. We applied a psychologically-based structure to his success story so that it could be told in a more meaningful manner to the business world. We had essentially teamed up as theorist and practitioner, and along with a third partner, Adrian Hutchinson, who provided the commercial experience and know-how, eventually set up a company called Lane4.

You and mental toughness

Lane4's work with some of the largest and best known companies in the UK over the past 12 years, and its recent expansion into North America and Australasia, reflects an enduring and worldwide demand that provides ample evidence of the power of applying the elite sporting metaphor to business. Numerous common factors across the two domains have already been identified, but one, in particular, stands out as fundamental to being successful in both – pressure. The highly visible and public nature of performance outcomes, together with the consequences of success and failure for performers in sport and business, mean that pressure is a huge factor in both worlds. The often fierce competition and the narrowest of margins that define success or failure mean that performers have to be able to cope with pressure.

Is merely *coping* with pressure sufficient to enable high performance to be delivered at a sustainable level? This book is underpinned by the key principle that high achievers do more than merely cope with pressure – they *thrive* on it! And the vital factor in thriving on pressure and moving to even higher levels of performance is the development of mental toughness.

Mental toughness lies at the core of the world's very best sports performers. It enables them to thrive on pressure that others find almost unbearable and merely cope as best they can. It builds and sustains a level of self-belief that makes their dreams become reality when others fall short because their belief isn't strong enough. It instills a motivation and determination in them to succeed when others are floored by failures and setbacks. It ensures an immovable focus when others are derailed by inevitable distractions. No wonder business executives have recently become enthralled and engrossed in the notion of mental toughness!

Over the last few years Adrian and I have been applying the elite sport metaphor with business executives to develop a level of mental toughness that enables them to deliver consistently high levels of performance under pressure. I have no doubt that you are reading this book because you, too, would like to deliver consistently high levels of performance under pressure. You may have already reached a high level in the corporate world and want to continue your development to achieve even greater things. Alternatively, you may have high potential and are looking for ways to aspire to your own and others' high expectations of you. For those of you who may be coaching or managing high achievers or high potentials, this book will serve as a valuable resource for supporting them when under pressure, and as an aid to their general personal development.

Content and layout of the book

The content of this book is designed to be thought-provoking, to raise awareness and to provide key pointers as to how you can develop and enhance your and others' mental toughness. The insights into mental toughness are based upon a number of different sources, specifically:

- my experiences of working with some of the world's best sport performers and their support staff;
- my experiences of working with performers at all levels of business organisations, including chief executive officers, managing directors and their boards;
- my experiences of working with elite performers in several other contexts, ranging from armed fighting force personnel to musicians;
- my published and ongoing research in the area of mental toughness and high level performance;
- my interpretation of the available theory and research findings in the area of performance psychology;
- Adrian's experiences of achieving World Number One status and sustaining it over six consecutive years;
- Adrian's transition from Olympic Gold Medallist to running a successful global company.

The book portrays a journey that begins with understanding why mental toughness is important, and what it actually is. Subsequent chapters then progress into how each of the elements of mental toughness can be developed and enhanced. Brief outlines of each chapter are as follows.

Chapter 2 highlights the enormous role played by pressure in both business and sport and draws parallels between them. It defines what pressure is and describes how it can debilitate your performance. Chapter 2 also describes how it is possible for you to thrive on pressure through the development of mental toughness.

Chapter 3 addresses what mental toughness is and what it is not, culminating in the identification of the four pillars of mental toughness:

- keeping your head under stress;
- staying strong in your self-belief;

- making your motivation work for you;
- maintaining your focus on the things that matter.

Chapter 4 deals with keeping your head under stress. It emphasises how understanding what stress is, and how it affects you, is the essential starting point. This chapter describes how the vast majority of stress is self-imposed and then presents three ways of keeping your composure under stress:

- managing the symptoms of stress;
- being able to control and change any negative thoughts;
- dealing with the source of stress itself.

Chapter 5 addresses the area of staying strong in your self-belief and how deep, inner belief enables you to deliver consistently high performance under pressure. This chapter distinguishes between self-esteem and self-confidence, and describes strategies and techniques for building both in order to develop and enhance a robust self-belief.

Chapter 6 reveals how making your motivation work for you is crucial in enabling you to remain motivated for the daily grind of work and also to recover from setbacks. This chapter distinguishes between different types of motivation and how some can actually debilitate performance under pressure. It examines what optimal motivation is and how to achieve it on a consistent basis.

Chapter 7 deals with the many potential distractions that you encounter and how maintaining your focus on the things that matter enables you to remain focused on key priorities when the pressure is really on. This chapter also describes how some situations require you to be able to switch your focus, often very rapidly. A number of strategies and techniques for enhancing both types of focus are described.

Chapter 8 concludes the book by addressing the questions I have been most frequently asked about mental toughness:

- What difference will it really make if I improve my mental toughness?
- Can you be too mentally tough?
- Just how easy is it to develop mental toughness?

- What about mental toughness in teams?
- How is mental toughness different from emotional intelligence?

The entire book includes a number of approaches and perspectives that make the topic of mental toughness easily accessible.

- Simple models and frameworks that illustrate the key components of the various elements of mental toughness.
- Stories about performers I have worked with that demonstrate how the core principles of mental toughness apply to 'real' business and sport performers.
- 'Over to Adrian' sections that bring alive key principles underlying mental toughness and its development.
- 'Time Out' sections that provide the opportunity to reflect and build on your growing awareness as you understand more about mental toughness and how you can develop and enhance it. To get the most out of the book do each Time Out as you come to it. I suggest you keep a notebook in which you can record your responses, together with any other thoughts and ideas you bring to mind whilst reading the book.
- 'In a Nutshell' sections in each chapter that summarise key messages.
- 'What Next?' sections at the end of chapters that deal with the four pillars of mental toughness that spell out actions that will help you develop and enhance each pillar.
- 'Case Studies' spanning the whole book that track the development of mental toughness in four performers.[2]

The book is designed with the intention that you can consult separate chapters for guidance on how to develop and enhance specific elements of mental toughness. However, you will benefit most from reading the book in its entirety and then keeping it close to hand as a continual reminder of how you can thrive on pressure.

---

[2] For the purpose of anonymity, the names used in any case illustrations are fictitious and certain details about all of the performers referred to in the book may have been altered. This is no way detracts from the key messages and authenticity of the references, stories and case studies.

2 Why Mental Toughness is Important

After reading this chapter you will know about:

- What pressure is, and its different sources
- How pressure can either facilitate or debilitate your performance
- How stress is a negative and often debilitating response to pressure

Having been involved with performers at World Championships, Olympic Games and World Cups on the one hand, and with business performers at the core of mergers, acquisitions, redundancies, management buyouts and flotations on the other, I have had first-hand experience of the enormous pressure that can both make and destroy people. I have witnessed people fold under pressure, and I have worked with people who thrive on it. Like it or not, in the arenas of business and sport, whether it be major events like those referred to above or the incessant daily demands of delivering consistent high level performance, pressure surrounds you and, sometimes, consumes you.

Over to Adrian . . .

In my swimming days there were numerous examples of performers wilting under the pressure of competition, and those who just seemed to 'step up'. On some occasions it was those closest to the performers who could have the most dramatic impact – the coach who became agitated and fidgety around swimmers just before the race, offering pearls of wisdom such as 'don't mess up your start!'

What is so pressured about sport and business?

I wouldn't have told it to a soul back then, but as early as my first Wimbledon in '77 I realised I had the potential to be the very best: the best tennis player in the world. I confirmed it for myself as I rose through the rankings – but then, more and more, the problem became that almost everybody was somebody I shouldn't lose to. The pressure became incomprehensible.

John McEnroe[3]

It doesn't take much to roll a 1.68 inch ball along a smooth, level surface into, or in the vicinity of, a 4.5 inch hole. With no pressure on you, you can do it one-handed most of the time. But there is always pressure on the shorter putts...90 per cent of the rounds I play in major championships, I play with a bit of a shake.

Jack Nicklaus[4]

Given that John McEnroe and Jack Nicklaus were at the very top of the world rankings during their careers in tennis and golf respectively, and are today legends in their own lifetimes, you could be forgiven for thinking that such superhumans would be immune to the pressure that can destroy mere mortals. As McEnroe and Nicklaus are acutely aware, pressure, and the ability to deal with it, was pretty important in their success. And this demand has, if anything, become even more prominent amongst modern day sporting icons:

It all went quiet. Everything was swirling around me, every nerve standing on edge. What's going on here? I can't breathe... I remember forcing in two big gulps of air to try and steady myself and take control...I was far too nervous to try to be clever. Not nervous for myself any longer. This was all about the team I was captain of. I've never felt such pressure before. I ran forward. And I kicked the ball goalwards as hard as I could...In.

David Beckham referring to his match-winning goal from a penalty kick in the crucial match against Argentina in the 2002 World Cup.[5]

---

[3] John McEnroe, *Serious: The Autobiography*, Penguin Putnam Inc, 2002, pp. 131–132.
[4] Jack Nicklaus with K.Bowden, *Golf My Way*, Pan, 1976, p .236.
[5] David Beckham, *My Side*, Collins Willow, 2003, pp. 273–274.

Sport at this level is more than just a game. Events such as the Olympic Games, the soccer World Cup, Wimbledon's tennis Grand Slam and the rugby World Cup are global media spectacles which attract huge audiences, and hence massive financial investment and potential profit. Take the 2003 rugby union World Cup final between Australia and England, for instance; an estimated three hundred million people worldwide watched the match on television, during which the traffic volume on British roads fell by 60 per cent and 37 million pints of beer were consumed in 10,000 British pubs that opened to screen the 9 am kick-off.[6] Sport is undeniably big business for the sponsors, the organisers and the performers themselves. Amongst headlines greeting the England team on their glorious return to home shores were some which even predicted a boost to the nation's economy as a result of their success.

Added to that is the fact that sport is so important in our culture that national prestige and identity are often heavily dependent on the success of our nation's sporting teams. On the morning after England's rugby victory over Australia, the British media were awash with how the nation's mood had been stunningly transformed. Prime Minister Tony Blair was quick to claim the victory as one not only for English rugby but for the whole of England too. French President Jacques Chirac even went so far as to claim it as a victory for Europe.

Over to Adrian . . .

In a similar way to the examples Graham has given, the impact of representing your nation can bring added pressure, even though it is a huge honour. At my second Olympics the racing followed a similar pattern to before, with the swimming events opening the Games. This meant that my race would be the first opportunity for a Gold Medal – not just for me but the entire Great Britain Olympic team. It wasn't until I read the press articles afterwards that I realised just how much had been placed on that result. Whether true or not, it seems as though I 'inspired the whole team to a great Olympics' by winning on that first day.

The lead-up to the final had provided an entertaining stage for nationalistic jousting and posturing. During the tournament the Australian press, clearly fearful of the threat posed by the England team to their own

6 Bryan Appleyard, 'Champions of the World', *The Sunday Times*, 23 November, 2003, p.1.

team's World Champions' crown, took it upon themselves to go far beyond the bounds of sporting decency in an attempt to taunt and humiliate not only the national rugby team but, ultimately, a whole nation. Even English 'jewels' such as *Coronation Street* and *Eastenders* were targets for Australian ridicule. And in a previous rugby World Cup, such was the importance of South Africa's success in the 1995 rugby final against New Zealand, after numerous years in the apartheid wilderness, that there was a significant level of curiosity over the number of All Black players who went down with food poisoning on the eve of the game.

There have been numerous instances over the years when the crossover between sport and other aspects of national culture and identity have reached sometimes preposterous proportions. An editorial in an English newspaper on the eve of the 1966 World Cup soccer final between England and the former West Germany attempted to convince readers that the game should be viewed as on a par with two world wars:

> *if, perchance, on the morrow, Germany should beat us at our own national game, let us take comfort from the fact that twice we have beaten them at theirs.*[7]

Cricket, too, has found itself at the centre of intense nationalistic passions. Going back as far as the 1932–33 Test Series between England and Australia, the infamous 'bodyline' controversy created a matter of national honour and identity in the form of a diplomatic dispute between the two nations. And the more recent 'Keating affair' only served to make any relationship founded on sporting links between the two nations even worse. The Australian Prime Minister had the audacity to place his hand on the Queen of England's royal personage in public! To add insult to injury, Keating's wife refused to curtsey to Her Majesty, and Keating then delivered a speech questioning his country's ties with Britain. The subsequent World Cup clash between Australia and England assumed a different mantle; this was definitely more than just a game. England's victory in that match, largely due to Ian Botham's performance, was greeted in the English media with emotions which extended far beyond the boundaries of sport. Headlines included *To Keating from Botham with Love* and *Oz-Zat: Royal Avenger Stuffs the Aussies*.[8] The British Prime Minister at the time, John Major, was also reported as interrupting

---

[7] J. Michener, *Sport in America*, Random House, New York, 1976, p. 427.

[8] Cited in: Joe Maguire, 'Globalisation, sport and national identities: The Empire Strikes Back', *Sport and Leisure*, 16, 1993, p. 303.

a cabinet meeting to announce the result. And any reference to England versus Australia cricket tussles will now always include reminiscences about the epic 2005 Test series which captured the hearts and minds of so many English men and women who not only didn't previously follow the game, but didn't know the rules either! Such was the whole nation's hunger for the much-awaited success over the Aussies.

Negative consequences of pressure

Such pressure to be successful can result in unacceptable consequences. One of America's leading medical experts, Dr Robert Goldman, surveyed 200 world-class athletes just before the 2000 Sydney Olympic Games and posed the far-reaching question: if there existed a pill that would make you unbeatable for the next five years, after which you would die – would you take it? Incredibly, 52 per cent responded in the affirmative![9] And recent drug scandals involving a number of world-class athletes who have tested positive for illegal performance-enhancing drugs reflect a continuing quest to win at all costs using the most unscrupulous methods imaginable.

Over to Adrian . . .

I was very aware of the efforts some of my competitors would make to try to win. Some were illegal and some downright dirty. Whilst never actually observing doping first-hand, one incident brought home to me just how desperate some of my rivals were. During the mid-80s the authorities were only just getting their act together with regards to doping (after all, this was prime achievement time for the East German swimming team!). At an open meeting in Monaco, previously never having any testing during racing, in between the prelims and finals they suddenly decided to introduce testing after each of the evening's finals. I subsequently turned up for the final to discover that only three others and myself were there for the race (out of eight qualified). I heard various excuses such as food poisoning, influenza, personal problems . . . and my favourite 'he slipped in the shower'.

---

[9] David Bond, 'A Battle Won, An Unwinnable War', *The Sunday Times*, 26 October, 2003, p. 2.14.

There are many more stories to tell like these that serve to demonstrate how much pressure is involved in top level sport. Indeed, high level performance and pressure are inseparable. Dominic Mahony, Bronze medallist in the modern pentathlon at the 1988 Olympic Games and Manager of the Great Britain pentathlon team at the 2000 Sydney and 2004 Athens Games, recently captured the intense pressure that performers experience:

> *I have just returned from a 'pressure-cooker' week away with the (GB) pentathlon team competing in the (2003) World Championships. It is the week of the year in which all the hopes and expectations of athletes and coaches come ruthlessly into focus. A test of whether people are ready to perform, whether they can cope . . . The pleasure of searching for the best in ourselves juxtaposed with disappointment and failure; an atmosphere of excitement and possibility juxtaposed with crushing pressure and dysfunctional behaviour. It was a humbling experience.*[10]

Mahony's quote says it all about the experience of performers at the highest level; the anticipation of the elation of achieving a dream conflicting with the fear that you might fail, and what that might bring; the see-saw of emotions and behaviours that will be experienced in the quest for that dream; digging deep within for meaning and resources that will help when things get tough; and, of course, the pressure that crushes, if you let it. And the world is full of spectators who will go to great lengths to watch all this unfold. There is nothing more exhilarating, tantalising and spellbinding than witnessing titanic tussles between evenly-matched opposition and the wondrous uncertainty that keeps fingernails short and bottoms gripping the edges of seats very tightly indeed.

Sport does not have exclusivity on pressure, of course. I have witnessed levels of pressure in some business organisations that would rival the most extreme levels in elite sport. And it's getting worse. We live in turbulent economic times, in which big companies are failing more frequently and performance slumps are proliferating. The uncertainty and apparent lack of full control over corporate destiny create enormous pressure.

There is a subtle difference, though, between sport and business in this respect. In sport, dealing with pressure is part of the 'test' that performers *choose* to participate in; however, in the business context this type of pressure is not something that most people would actually choose to

---

[10] Dominic Mahony, *Steel and Shadow; An Inquiry into the Nature of Competition*, unpublished M.A. Dissertation, 2003, p. 2.

subject themselves to. Instead, it is often an unwanted distracter, and sometimes detractor, from individual, team and organisational performance. And the consequences of failure are potentially more catastrophic at the personal level, with redundancy, demotion, severance, burnout and ill health lurking around the corner.

The pressures on leaders

I have been particularly intrigued by my experiences of working with leaders in both sport and business organisations. It has been fascinating to compare the demands on managing directors and chief executive officers with those of head coaches of high profile sports teams. These are the people held responsible and accountable for the performance of organisations and teams; they get sacked and hired based on their people's performances. There is no hiding place for leaders at this level. As depicted in Figure 2.1, their job is to establish a clear vision for the organisation and to formulate a strategy that will deliver that vision. The vision and strategy must then be communicated to the whole organisation. As part of this process, the leader must exhibit a level of rational thinking sufficient to satisfy some and convince others that logic has prevailed. In communicating the vision and strategy, the leader also needs to exhibit the emotional side of him or herself which will inspire everyone to follow.

Figure 2.1 No hiding place for leaders.

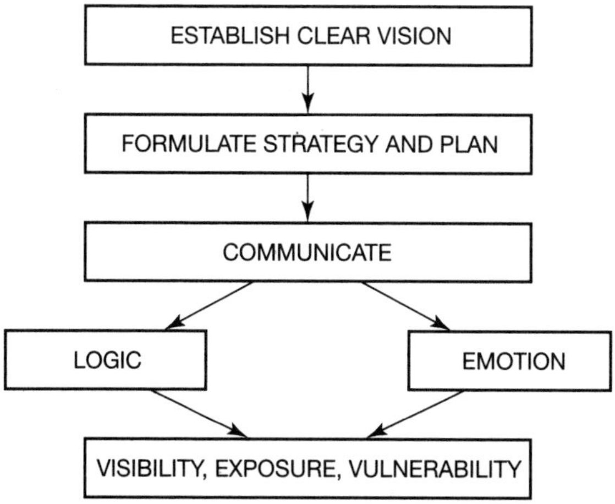

This whole process makes leaders highly visible, exposed and vulnerable. So much so that many of the people I have worked with at the highest levels of business and sport leadership are so continuously visible and exposed that they sometimes feel isolated and lonely. They are sometimes unable to identify who their true friends and allies are.

Sadly, I have witnessed situations in which leaders have succumbed to the intense pressure they have experienced. Two specific cases come to mind.

Case studies

Chris

The first involved Chris, a highly intelligent man and a successful and well-respected coach who cared very much for his players and the team's support staff. He was also highly visible. He coached a team that figured in the national newspapers in some form or another most days of the week. He enjoyed wide acclaim and hero status in a 'love affair' with the team's fans. His team was successful, he was his own man and he did things his way. Alas, things began to go wrong. The team spiralled into a seemingly unassailable losing run. Previously friendly media turned into bloodthirsty critics. Chris stopped reading the newspapers. He stopped shopping in the local supermarket - the open abuse was intolerable.

As the losing run grew longer, he succumbed to the pundits' cries for popular selections - he was no longer his own man. Chris felt exposed, highly vulnerable and lonely. He began to ask me what the newspapers were saying about him, what people thought of him. Chris would deliver a rousing team talk just before a game and then retire to the stand to become one of tens of thousands of people who would witness whether he had done a good job or not. He was responsible for his team's performance but was virtually helpless once the contest began.

I had embarked on this adventure anticipating that I would be heavily involved with the team - I spent most of my time supporting Chris and caring for his well-being. He visited me in my hotel room the morning after one particularly painful defeat and asked if he should resign. The pressure was on and Chris had lost sight of how to deal with it. He had lost his motivation to carry on - he was too focused on the things that were going wrong, and he had lost belief in himself and his undoubted ability as a coach.

Andy

The second case is that of Andy, a newly-appointed managing director of a large division of a well-known global company. A mutual friend who knew of my work in the area of mental toughness put us in contact, informing me that Andy was quite clearly stressed about work. I called Andy to arrange our first meeting and he was very keen that our 'liaison' should be a closely kept secret; after all, a managing director should be able to cope ▶

with pressure! In that first meeting, Andy talked at length about the huge expectations on him, and his loneliness and vulnerability based around his own perceptions that colleagues who were overlooked when he was appointed were just waiting for him to fail.

The root of it all was Andy's belief that he had been fortunate to get the position, that there were people more experienced and qualified to do the job. He was just waiting for them to find him out. In essence, it was his lack of self-belief that was causing the problem and this was exacerbated when the pressure was really on. His focus on how lucky he was became even more pronounced, and he loathed presenting to his board members and other colleagues on relatively mundane issues. His motivation became more to do with avoiding failure.

These two cases encapsulate the enormous pressure that leaders in both sport and business often endure. I'm sure you will be glad to know that both Chris and Andy came to learn how to deal with their respective circumstances via a number of different strategies and techniques described later in this book. Their development of mental toughness will be tracked in case studies that follow in subsequent chapters.

→ Business pressures

The pressure to perform in business extends beyond leaders, of course, with modern day executives facing numerous challenges. Factors such as globalisation, rapid technological changes, labour market deregulation, shifts in employment patterns and changes in organisational structures have all played a part in influencing career patterns. With increased globalisation, often accompanied by organisational restructuring, comes the need for cost competitiveness, high innovation and quality. This globalisation has demanded communication technology advances to ensure the rapid transmission of information. Technological advances in other areas have meant the automation of previously labour-intensive processes, particularly in manufacturing. Labour market deregulation means reduced job security, and with it the need to regularly update skills and knowledge in the context of fewer opportunities for lifelong employment. In sometimes desperate attempts to adapt to the pressures of change, organisations are continually restructuring, sometimes in the form of downsizing and delayering, resulting in fewer opportunities for promotion and, when they do occur, the jumps tend to be greater in terms of increased responsibility. Decentralising, merging and even upsizing are other options open to organisations, but whatever the chosen path, employees are increasingly faced with disruption to their working lives.

With all of this comes the pressure to manage the 'soft' side of people well; their motivation, their confidence, their personalities. Managers now have the added pressure of managing people rather than merely managing the completion of tasks. Managing people is hard. They have their own views on how things should be done. They have feelings and emotions, which are sometimes unpredictable, unexpected and inexplicable. They have frailties and make mistakes. They like to be praised and to be made to feel good about themselves. Put simply, this humanistic management drive is placing even more demands on managers and leaders; they are now being asked to be coaches too!

Over to Adrian . . .

For me some of the key similarities and differences in sport and business pressures are:

Similarities: performing whilst fatigued; the pressure of winning a race/sales pitch; the influence of a coach/leader's behaviours, whether it be good or bad; the distractions of others (less committed) in training/the office.

Differences: there is more real physical pain in sport, which can add to the fear of what is about to happen. Also, Graham's point about having the choice, the intrinsic desire to actually *be* in that Olympic final, or that Cup Final (should you be talented enough to be able to get there in the first place) is more real for sports people. I do believe, however, that in business people have more control over what happens to them than they think.

Worse still, workers are not the only ones affected by pressure; their families are also often at risk. Trade unions, recognising that their members' priorities have changed from traditional, old-fashioned wage disputes, are now focusing more and more on work-life balance issues emanating within the modern 'work-till-you-drop' culture. Life coaches have never been so evident or so popular.

What is pressure?

It will have become evident in the previous section that pressure assumes many forms and guises that can be most easily explained and understood by considering the relationship between you and the environment you operate in. The most obvious and common sources are those imposed on you by the environment (see 'a' in Figure 2.2), such as lack of time, uncertainty, high expectations, lack of control, constant change, high visibility, making difficult choices and competition. These externally-imposed pressures are often seen and accepted as 'part of the territory', and almost certainly increase the further up the corporate ladder you climb. For Chris, the coach referred to in the previous section, the external pressures had started to overwhelm him. He was attempting to deliver against the enormous, and unrealistic, expectations of the numerous stakeholders who closely observed and commented on his every move.

There is another very important source of pressure that is probably not quite so obvious – yourself! You are often your own worst enemy. Think back to a recent 'performance': a presentation, a competition, a sales pitch, an interview, a meeting you chaired. What were the sources of pressure? How many were completely imposed on you and outside your control? More importantly, how much pressure did you put on yourself?

Self-imposed pressure essentially takes two forms. The first is pressure that you actually seek out in the external environment (see 'b' in Figure 2.2). An extreme example is the sensation-seeker who goes to great lengths to experience the thrill and adrenaline-pumping excitement of activities such as bungee jumping, off-piste skiing, parachuting, placing large spread betting stakes and the like. At a less extreme, more 'normal' level, most people seek pressures that make their day-to-day existence more interesting and challenging. These will vary enormously between individuals, but can include setting stretching goals, aspiring to the next promotion, studying for that next qualification, etc. Pressure in this latter form essentially reflects your own personal ambitions, and results from choices you have made about how you want to live your life and what you wish to achieve during it.

Figure 2.2 Where does pressure come from?

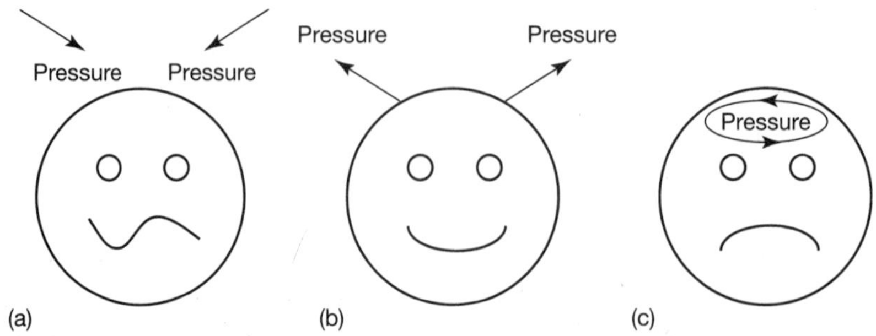

You don't always have the same level of control over the second type of self-imposed pressure – that cunning form that lives inside your head (see 'c' in Figure 2.2). This sometimes assumes the guise of a monster that plays games with your mind and creates pressure when it shouldn't exist. It plays with your conscience and distorts your perceptions of reality. It turns molehills into mountains. It sees problems when there are none. It creates high expectations that are not actually expected. The more deep-seated version of this monster lies in aspects of your personality. The pessimists and perfectionists amongst you will understand this much better than the optimists and realists and will know immediately what I mean! I will return to this later in the book.

For Andy, the managing director referred to in the previous section, much of his pressure was self-imposed – he had done a wonderful job of conjuring up enormous pressure in his own mind. His perceptions that 'he was lucky to be in the position' and that 'there were people working for him who were better for the job' led to further distorted expectations that he believed he could never deliver against.

At other times, when you are in control of your thoughts and emotions, this form of self-imposed pressure can be harnessed and used to turn everyday, often monotonous activities into learning experiences and opportunities to develop strategies to cope with and thrive on pressure when it really does exist. Practising penalty kicks in training under self-imposed, simulated pressure conditions provides an example from sport, and might have helped England soccer players cope better with the pressure cauldron of penalty shoot-outs in high profile competitions over the last few years. Similarly, building that weekly departmental presentation into something bigger than it actually is, so that coping strategies can be practised for that big presentation to the board next month, is an example from business of self-imposed pressure being employed, in a controlled manner, to aid personal development.

Over to Adrian . . .

The main pressure that I had as a swimmer came from myself. Of course, the fact that I was in the environment of the Olympic Games was in itself a pressure, but I had sought it out, and so in that regard it was self-imposed. I liked the challenge of racing and as I competed more internationally I enjoyed the more thrilling races. Where it became a bit too much was in my first Olympics when I started to magnify all the implications of what losing might be, letting down my parents, letting down my coach.

Before the 1984 Games, reading the headline 'Wilkie '76, Goodhew '80, Moorhouse '84?' alluding to the expectation that I would be the third British breaststroke Gold Medal winner in consecutive Olympics, caused me to distort the impact of winning or losing. My mind started playing tricks on me, and it became the most important thing in my life. This caused a lot of pressure of a type that I was unable to deal with.

In 1988 things were very different. In many ways this was down to maturity, and the capacity to think about challenges and life in a more philosophical way. I had realised that it was important to keep things in perspective. It was, after all, just a swimming race. It didn't take me long to think of people in situations that could rightly be considered more challenging than mine. Besides, what a great opportunity to really race the other swimmers on a big stage. I also thought that some of them were probably scared of me now!

Right now as Managing Director of Lane4, I enjoy being in the business and the thrill of entrepreneurship; it has been very exciting being involved in starting a company from scratch, and now 12 years on, in building a thriving business. But this role brings other pressures, such as making big decisions, something that was still true as a swimmer, but a key decision about financial investments is a bit different from wondering which trunks to wear. I also find myself trying to balance time at work with my commitments to my family – nothing new for most people with a family who also work – but so hard to do, particularly if expecting a conference call from the United States at 8pm. In reality, I find myself with more of a similar role to that of my coach – managing a team of performers with all their various idiosyncrasies!

So pressure takes at least two forms: pressure that is externally-imposed and pressure that is self-imposed by either actively seeking it in the environment or through creation of pressure within your own mind. You are likely to be subjected to, and subject yourself to, all forms at various points in time. So how do you respond when you are under these different pressures? Are you aware of being under pressure? What thoughts, feelings and behaviours characterise your response? How do you perform?

Pressure tends to bring out the chameleon in all of us. At its worst, pressure can make the human existence miserable and unbearable, resulting in high levels of stress[11] that debilitate your performance. At its best, pressure can enrich your life, making it fulfilling and meaningful, inspiring you to higher, and even extraordinary, levels of performance. The essence of this book lies in the proposition that how you experience pressure and how it affects you is largely your own choice. It may not seem like it sometimes, but you do not have to be stressed and debilitated by pressure. In fact you can positively thrive on it!

→ Do only the tough survive?

Why do some tennis players succumb to the pressure of playing in their first Wimbledon final and others look like they belong there? Why do some performers love the pressure of being involved in penalty shootouts and others curl up at the very thought of them? Why do some traders lose self-confidence and motivation after a dramatic trading loss, and others come back stronger and more determined? The simple fact is that we are all different and respond differently to pressure.

Case studies

Scott and Emma are examples of performers I have worked with that reflect just how big a factor pressure can be in impairing performance.

Scott

Scott was fulfilling his lifelong dream – playing as a professional golfer on the European Tour. As a young amateur, he had been tipped for great things and he lived for his chosen sport. Midway through his first year as a professional he was struggling to make cuts, let alone appear on the leader ▶

[11] The distinction between 'pressure' and 'stress' will be addressed at length in Chapter 4. For the time being, stress should be viewed as a negative and potentially debilitative reaction to pressure.

board going into final rounds. It looked like Scott wouldn't keep his card for the following year. The enjoyment factor had disappeared; his sport was now his job and he depended on it for his and his new wife's financial security. As tournaments came and went, and his debts continued to mount, the almost intolerable pressure was producing stress levels that were affecting both his performance and his life. He was plagued by uncertainty and feeling out of control. His confidence was at rock bottom. Scott needed success fast, and the more he needed success, the less successful he became. He was beginning to hate the sport he loved.

Emma

Emma was keen to emphasise in our first meeting that she was a woman holding a senior position in a male-dominated environment. She was acutely aware of a need to perform, not simply because she had a position of responsibility, but also because she was female. All eyes were on Emma; every word she spoke in meetings with her male colleagues was under the closest scrutiny – at least, that's what she thought! I'm sure that there was something in what she was telling me. Her male colleagues probably *were* very interested in her performance, but more as a functional director than as a female. Emma was feeling the pressure of being a woman rather than a director, and was trying to be somebody and something else in the presence of her colleagues – she was certainly not being the individual who had been appointed to her position. Emma's motivation to succeed was founded on a self-imposed pressure that had a negative underpinning; she perceived that her male colleagues thought she was not good enough for the job and she wanted to prove them wrong. Fired by this intense need, her judgements, decision making and behaviour became impaired and distorted – she was self-destructing.

I have drawn on the examples of Scott and Emma not only to illustrate how pressure can debilitate performance, but also to emphasise that it is possible to turn these situations around. Using the strategies and techniques addressed later in this book, Scott managed to keep his card and in the next season figured on leader boards with players who had previously served as sources of inspiration to him – Nick Faldo, Colin Montgomerie, Fred Couples, Ernie Els and the like. Emma was eventually able to perceive herself as a director of a company, rather than as a woman in a male-dominated environment, and this enabled her to approach her job from a very different perspective and demonstrate her true capability. Scott's and Emma's development of mental toughness will be tracked along with coach, Chris, and managing director, Andy, in '**C**hris **A**ndy **S**cott **E**mma Studies' described in subsequent chapters.

The fact that some performers are seriously debilitated in pressured environments is openly exploited in the sporting world. The attempts in recent years to outlaw 'sledging' (the verbal abuse of batsmen from the fielding side) in cricket illustrates that this exploitation can be one of the less appealing sides to sport. The great Australian side under their former captain, Steve Waugh, openly referred to a policy of 'mental disintegration' to root out the psychologically weak amongst their opponents. And in football's Premiership League in England, the frequent wars of words and apparent hostility played out in the media between managers of teams competing for the top prizes are often attempts to heap even more pressure on to their opponents. Sir Alex Ferguson, Jose Mourinho, Arsene Wenger and occasionally some other managers who fancy their chances in the psyche-out arena provide an entertaining sideshow to the pressures played out on the field.

Over to Adrian . . .

Mental toughness in swimming is absolutely crucial, and I do believe it's the same in business. I started to understand it after I lost the Olympics in '84. I realised that most things affecting my preparation and performance were in my control. Something I had to develop the most after that defeat was an understanding of where my self-belief came from. When I stood up for a race I did get excited about competing against the best in the world, whereas before I would worry that they would be better than me. I just concentrated on all my strengths and enjoyed just getting amongst it. I would always swim faster than I could in training, I almost needed the pressure of racing to stretch myself.

There were a number of examples of swimmers who were very talented, but couldn't quite cope with the pressures of competing. One particular swimmer I knew would train extremely hard, but seem to throw it away at the big events. For example, after months of training twice a day (with 5 o'clock starts each day), in the last week of competition I would see him doing things slightly out of the ordinary – late nights, drinking, smoking etc!

There was also a Russian swimmer, a competitor of mine, who I raced frequently between 1985 and 1992, who would always get the Bronze or Silver behind me. Now, I don't know whether he started off believing he could beat me, but I certainly remember the time when he stopped – at the European Championships in 1989. After winning the Olympics in 1988 I broke my wrist and didn't swim for a long time – over four months. I think he thought I had quit as I didn't race him for most of 1989. So when I turned up at the European Championships in Bonn I remember seeing him looking more confident than he had ever looked before, but surprised to see me. Then in the heats I broke the World Record and he collapsed . . . and I saw the look on his face, and I think it was a collapse of his mental toughness.

In business, we are in a competitive world, particularly in our sector, yet I am not afraid of failing. For me it is more about working on our strengths and recognising we have a lot to offer the market. A lot of the time it is about not being distracted by other people and their pessimism, but staying true to your strategy and silencing the negative voices – even if they are in your own head!

This test of mental strength is also a core part of the world of business at its most ruthless. Chivalry and valour are usually low on the list of priorities in organisations desperately striving for market share in an ailing economic climate. With job security and career progression often uncertain, competing with colleagues can be a big factor in employees' daily working lives. Some people may feel they aren't cut out for the ruthlessness that may sometimes be required. They wilt under the pressure, often disillusioned and resentful of the fact that they find themselves in this position. For others, the incessant demand to hit targets which may be at best very stretching and, at worst, completely unattainable, will eventually wear them down. And all this occurs in the knowledge that there are others eager to step into their shoes at the first sign of weakness.

→ Thriving on pressure

In contrast, some performers are able to cope very well and even thrive in high pressure situations. Some business performers will relish the challenge of competing against their colleagues; some cricket batsmen will actually enjoy being on the receiving end of sledging. Steve Backley, former javelin World Record holder and Olympic Medallist, in an interview for a research study I carried out a number of years ago, described how pressure was a very positive factor for him, estimating that it improved his performance by as much as ten per cent in competition when compared with training. This helps to explain the numerous times Backley came through the field to achieve medal positions with his very last throw.

What is it about these performers that enables them to respond in this way? The answer is mental toughness. More than ability, more than experience, more than education, in today's fast-moving, highly competitive world, it is a person's level of mental toughness that will determine who succeeds and who fails. That's the case in the Olympics and it's true in the workplace.

Mental toughness enables you to bounce back after setbacks, to maintain belief in yourself when doubts are gnawing away at you, to remain focused in the face of numerous unwanted distractions, to keep going when all seems lost, to turn threats into opportunities, to find ways of motivating yourself when you are struggling to keep going, to harness thoughts and feelings so that they work for you rather than against you, to make choices when there appear to be none available, to remain in control and to even enjoy pressure. The good news is that mental toughness can be developed so that you too can learn to cope with and actually thrive on pressure.

In a nutshell

- Pressure can be broken down into externally-imposed and self-imposed sources.
- Externally-imposed pressures are those emanating from the environment, often in the form of others' expectations of you, constant change, uncertainty, etc.
- Self-imposed pressure takes two forms:
  1. pressure that you seek out in the environment, mainly in terms of choosing to put yourself in pressured situations;
  2. pressure that you bring upon yourself by distorting perceptions of reality and creating pressure in your own mind.
- Pressure can either facilitate or debilitate performance, depending on how you respond to it.
- Stress is a negative and often debilitating response to pressure.
- Mental toughness enables you to cope with and even thrive on pressure.

3 What Mental Toughness is

After reading this chapter you will know about:

- What mental toughness is
- What mental toughness is not
- The four pillars of mental toughness

I described in Chapter 2 how mental toughness is the key to delivering sustainable high levels of performance under pressure. However, I didn't actually provide a definition of this well-used but little understood concept. This chapter addresses what mental toughness is and what it isn't.

→ 'I need to be mentally tough, but what is it'?

Take a few moments to think about and identify elite sport performers who have demonstrated extraordinary mental toughness. I would be surprised if the name Steve Redgrave, five times Olympic rowing champion, didn't figure prominently in your list. People who rowed with him remember that he used to fall out of the boat with exhaustion in training, just to experience true pain, so that when a boat came back at him in a big race he knew that if he was hurting his opponent must be really suffering. Redgrave knew there was nobody as mentally strong as him out there.

However, mental toughness is not the exclusive property of the world's best performers. Think of someone *you* know in person who is mentally tough. Now consider what it is about this person that leads you to believe that he or she is mentally tough. Finally, how do you think or know he or she has developed this mental toughness?

Having posed these questions to numerous audiences, I have noticed a consistent pattern in their responses. They tend to have a general feel for what mental toughness is and how it might have been developed, but they have difficulty in pinpointing exactly what it is. Likewise, sports journalists and television and radio commentators invariably refer to the importance of mental toughness in determining sporting outcomes, but equally invariably, it is used to embrace a multitude of things that are never actually identified or defined. This is perhaps not so surprising since mentally tough, top level performers themselves often struggle to conjure up the words that accurately capture what their own mental toughness is. Their difficulty in verbalising and articulating what mental toughness is reflects something that is, or has become, innate in them; it effectively represents implicit rather than explicit knowledge.

The need for mental toughness

This lack of clarity around mental toughness is unfortunate, because it is often an expected but unwritten requirement for succeeding in high pressure environments. The business world is full of people in highly pressured jobs that demand mental toughness as the foundation of their success. Recovering from setbacks, dealing with difficult people, coping with change and uncertainty and missing targets are just a few of the potential sources of pressure that test the mettle of business performers.

It has also been fascinating to work with elite armed force recruits for whom mental toughness can eventually mean the difference between life and death. In fact, their training is essentially about sifting out those who do not possess the required mental strength to deal with this extreme of pressure. Those who can't hack the incredible physical demands and public humiliation they are subjected to in the event of failure are slowly, and sometimes quickly, broken down and ousted. The gruelling, unrelenting hardship they are exposed to is an incessant test of their mental toughness. For some recruits, this experience will help to build their mental toughness, for others it can batter them into submission.

These situations and environments are all clearly observable examples of the need to be mentally tough. If you are mentally tough, then you possess the essential foundation of success; if not, then you run the risk of failing or never putting yourself on the line. A fundamental issue with this is that people are seldom supported and shown how to develop their mental toughness. This is a reflection of the fact that although mental toughness is extremely important and is even demanded of people, there has simply not been enough information and knowledge around about what it is and how to develop it.

What mental toughness is not

Following the publication of a study on mental toughness carried out by myself and co-researchers[12] (described in the next section), I was interviewed by a freelance journalist who was keen to explore the extent to which the findings applied to leaders in the business world. I was later dismayed to read the conclusions that had been drawn from the published research and subsequent interview when his article appeared in a well-circulated management journal. The article, entitled *If you think you're HARD enough*, raised my research to heady heights it has never been subjected to before – *This month MT (Management Today) can exclusively reveal new research on some of life's winners that will cause Dr Goleman* (author of the best seller *Emotional Intelligence*[13]) *and his followers to rethink their theories on touchy-feely management'*.[14] The article went on to suggest that my research pointed to the need for driven, leather-skinned bosses with no room for vulnerability and weakness. Worse still, alongside the text was a cartoon character representing a cross between Superman and Popeye with briefcase in hand, bulging muscles, a heavily tattooed torso and an aggressive facial expression. This image, together with the claim that *Nice guys don't finish first*, pointed to mental toughness as being characterised by such personal attributes as physical and mental hardness, masculinity, ruthlessness, defiance, stubbornness, lack of awareness and other similarly worrying associations.

In a similar vein, people eager to share with me their stories of mental toughness have often misconstrued its essential elements: 'did you hear about the footballer who played through the pain of a broken leg for the last ten minutes of a match?'; 'I know this senior executive who can go for three days without sleep when the pressure's really on to deliver'. Far from being dazzled and impressed by these apparent feats of 'mental toughness', I gently question the wisdom of such acts.

---

12 Graham Jones, Sheldon Hanton & Declan Connaughton. What is this thing called mental toughness? An investigation of elite performers. *Journal of Applied Sport Psychology*, 14, 205–218, 2002.

13 Daniel Goleman, *Emotional Intelligence*, Bantam Books, 1995.

14 Stefan Stern, 'If you think you're HARD enough', *Management Today*, March 2003, p. 4.

Case studies

A couple of real-life examples will help to clarify what mental toughness is not.

Kellee

Kellee was ranked number two in the world in a sport demanding quick reactions, power, agility and endurance. I had been working closely with her for over a year and we had devoted a significant amount of time to psychological skills that helped her to shut out negative thoughts and doubts during matches. These had helped Kellee to win the World Championship for the first and only time after many thwarted attempts. She still had another three or four good years in her when she sustained a niggling injury in training. She shouldn't have played in the next tournament, but she ignored the advice of the people around her. The injury was becoming worse and she continued to train and play in tournaments. I realised that Kellee was employing the techniques I had taught her to shut out negative thoughts to, instead, shut out the pain from her injury. She was putting short-term gains ahead of longer term aspirations and was, within a few months, forced to retire because her body was giving up on her. Kellee's ability to play through the pain may, at first sight, appear to reflect mental toughness; instead, it represented a weakness to focus only on the short-term that ended in the sacrifice of her longer term goals.

Ben

In another context, a very hard-working senior executive, Ben, whom I had got to know very well, finally succumbed to the ridiculous hours he was working when a virus forced him to consult a doctor. Routine tests unexpectedly showed the possibility of cancer, but he had to endure another two months' uncertainty before further tests could be carried out to enable an accurate diagnosis. Ben decided that there was no point in worrying, and chose to tell only his wife and no one else, including his grown-up children. He thought he was dealing with it very well as the important retest results got closer. He sat calmly with his wife in the consultant's waiting room until the fateful moment arrived. The consultant gave Ben the good news that it had been a virus and that he did not have cancer. Ben's wife became very emotional – he was numb! He had suppressed his emotions to such an extent that they were still squashed. What should have been an ecstatic moment was merely what felt like an 'emotionless' experience where even relief struggled to surface.

Ben spent the next few months completely drained and unable to deliver against his high expectations at work or home. He had suffered in silence, choosing not to seek support and to deny the existence of the problem and the support he so desperately needed. This was not mental toughness; instead, it was a complete lack of awareness of how to deal with a difficult situation.

Over to Adrian . . .

Leading up to 1984, I found myself in a similar position to the one Graham describes in the case study of Kellee, in that I was so driven by my goal to win the Olympics that I ignored some very obvious signs that I was overtraining – getting colds that I couldn't shake off, and taking longer than usual to recover from a hard weights session. I pushed on through because I thought that I couldn't miss any training. Instead, I became more tired as my body struggled to cope. In the end I entered the last few weeks before the Games in a very jaded state. This was mental weakness really, as the strong thing to do would have been to just rest for a couple of weeks earlier in the season when the initial signs were there.

Kellee and Ben highlight that one of the problems in using the sporting analogy to characterise mental toughness is that it tends to be associated with the absolute extremes of human endeavour. The earlier reference to Steve Redgrave is a prime example; mental toughness is often equated with things like pushing yourself to the limit and enduring extreme hardship. The natural assumption can be that mental toughness requires a 'hardness' that is associated with the less attractive side of human nature. Sure, some mentally tough people may not be individuals you would want to have a beer with, but so are other people who may *not* be mentally tough. My experience of working with mentally tough performers from different arenas is that they are, in fact, often open, fair-minded, caring and decent people.

Over to Adrian . . .

Showing others how hard and mentally tough you are seemed important to some swimmers I knew. An example I have is of somebody I used to train with. He would always come to the training sessions appearing quite aggressive with very little room for conversation or relaxed banter. He seemed to be pushing people away, in a very male way ('I don't need anyone, I'm really tough'). But whenever he was in any racing situation I could see him getting more and more flustered and he didn't seem to have the resources inside to cope. He also didn't want to accept any support from others. He was a really bad racer and wasn't able to perform. It was almost as if he had built up a shell around himself for the outside world, but didn't really know how to cope internally. It was his version of being 'tough', without any of the substance behind it. I have seen this many times in business. The truly mentally tough are actually quite rounded individuals.

Mental toughness is not, therefore, about ruthless, uncaring, hard-nosed, leather-skinned bosses with nerves of steel. Mental toughness is not about playing football through the excruciating pain of a broken leg, or the ability to voluntarily endure three nights without sleep – that is commonly known as stupidity! And it is certainly not exclusive to males or masculinity. So what is mental toughness?

→ What mental toughness is

My early research interest in stress and its effects upon performance was fuelled by a personal, incredibly frustrating confusion as to why I seldom produced my performance potential in highly pressurised sporting environments. Alas, the solution to the confusion came too late to satisfy my own sporting aspirations, but ignited an intense interest in the psychological make-up of elite performers. As I and my fellow researchers at Loughborough University conducted study after study into how sport performers respond to the pressure of competition, a clear pattern began to emerge in terms of key differences between 'elite' and 'good' performers.

Essentially, good performers reported their pre-performance heightened mental (e.g. apprehension, excitement, doubt) and physical (e.g. butterflies, heart rate, nausea, muscle tension, nervous) states as being relatively debilitative to their upcoming performance; elite performers, on the other hand, reported the same states as being facilitative.

This, to me, was a clear indication of mental control amongst the elite performers that constituted one important aspect of mental toughness. My recent research activities with Professor Sheldon Hanton and Declan Connaughton at the University of Wales Institute, Cardiff, have been targeted specifically at getting to grips with this thing called 'mental toughness'. This is a difficult concept to study because mentally tough performers themselves have difficulty verbalising and articulating something that is so implicit within them. For this reason, there has been very little worthwhile scientific research in the area.

Rising to the challenge Sheldon, Declan and I embarked on a programme of work aimed at defining mental toughness and identifying the key attributes that underpin it. Whilst this work initially looked at sport performers, studies currently being conducted within Lane4 in commercial organisations are reinforcing the transferability of these findings into the business performance arena.

The pillars of mental toughness

The model shown in Figure 3.1 was originally generated from studies involving elite performers who were asked to identify what mental toughness meant to them, and how it is manifested in other elite performers whom they considered to be particularly mentally tough. This model has been greeted with universal approval across the different performance arenas I have operated in. It has helped sport performers, in particular, understand a previously indeterminable but much needed psychological attribute. And performers in the business world have been able to make almost instant connections with what is required to sustain high levels of performance in their pressured environments. Indeed, it has been the cornerstone of one particular intervention with a company undergoing very significant change as the result of an acquisition.

Figure 3.1 The four pillars of mental toughness.

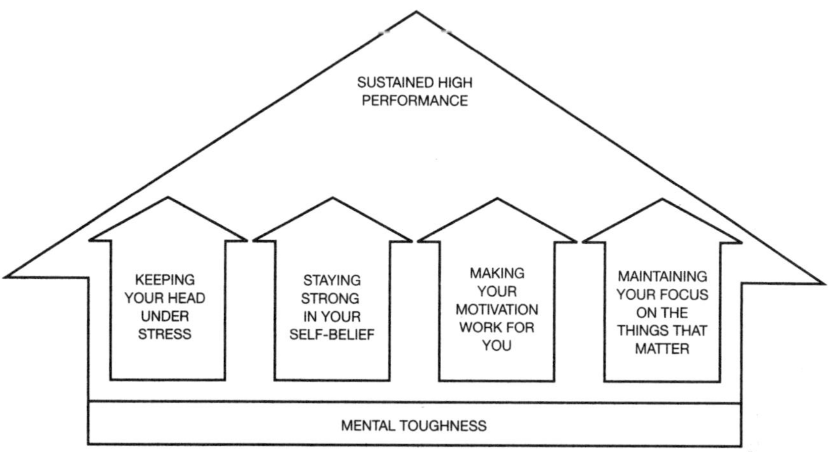

Mental toughness comprises four 'pillars' that form the foundation of sustained high performance – 'keeping your head under stress', 'making your motivation work for you', 'staying strong in your self-belief'and 'keeping focused on the things that matter'. These have been specifically identified in our studies of elite performers, and comprise the following:

- **Keeping your head under stress** – this pillar addresses the stress that can result from pressure and has the function of controlling the amount and nature of the stress you are under so that you can remain composed in weighing up the situation and making important decisions.

- **Staying strong in your self-belief** – this pillar has the function of providing the source of robust belief and confidence in your qualities and abilities required to achieve your performance goals.
- **Making your motivation work for you** – the function of this pillar is to ensure your desire and determination to succeed is founded on positive and constructive motives that keep you optimally motivated and enable you to recover from performance setbacks that may threaten your longer term goals.
- **Maintaining your focus on the things that matter** – the function of this pillar is to regulate your focus so that the many demands you encounter do not distract you from key priorities.

Over to Adrian . . .

I actually find it quite hard to articulate what mental toughness is. Some of it I am sure has been inside me from a very young age, but I am equally certain that getting through the various ups and downs in my life have contributed a large amount of learning. The four pillars that Graham describes help me to make sense of the various aspects of mental toughness that underpinned my success as a swimmer. As a framework, it also helps me to understand the core demands on me as a Managing Director and how I respond to them.

Keeping your head under stress - one area of pressure in my working life seems to be the overloaded diary. I look at the week ahead, and wonder not only how all these appointments got in there (usually my own fault), but also how I might actually make it through and maintain my sanity and health. The short-term solution is to take one day at a time - simple to say, harder to do. I am aware that I can compartmentalise things in my head quite well, and just seem to put the rest of the week away in a box, and concentrate on what is in front of me. It's the working equivalent of 'get the dive right', rather than 'beat the world'.

Staying strong in your self-belief - in my job now I still find myself making presentations in front of large groups of people. For the most part the audience is a peer group of HR professionals. In stepping up to talk I draw on many past experiences of things that I feel good about - and specifically related to the task in hand - not just my past swimming life!

Making your motivation work for you - I often get feedback that one of my strengths is a strong drive, or motivation to succeed. This has been a feature of my approach to things for as long as I can remember. I can only think that it was part of the values that ►

my parents brought to my brother's upbringing and mine. They were very strong role models – with my father being 'self made', having left school at 14. There was a clear message of personal responsibility for anything you wanted to achieve, and a strong work ethic. Having trained really hard for swimming in my early years, and seeing some success (even though at that point it was just the Bradford and District championships) I had evidence. Just get on and do it!

Maintaining your focus on the things that matter – again, another one easier to say than actually do. I think that it does help if you have broken down the big goal into smaller, manageable chunks. I occasionally found myself in training thinking about winning races, but it was obvious to me that it was a waste of time really. I had to get on with tackling the specific objectives that would build up to make me a great swimmer – then winning races would be more likely. Another distraction nowadays at work is the never-ending stream of emails that seem to arrive just when I am concentrating on writing a paper or proposal. I have created small strategies for that, such as turning off the notification noises, or even shutting down the computer.

The four pillars of mental toughness will be addressed in detail in Chapters 3 to 6. For the time being, Libby and Jack's stories below exemplify the four pillars and how they are enacted in real life.

Case studies

Libby

Libby had just attained official World Number One status and was under enormous pressure to do the 'celebrity thing' and cash in on her success. Libby had other ideas. She was not about to let short-term gains distract her from her longer-term goals. She would celebrate her success accordingly but then re-focus on staying ahead of the opposition and setting standards the sport had never seen before. Libby was being mentally tough, withstanding the external pressures, re-focusing on the things that had kept her motivated during the long, sometimes gruelling and painful hours of training and preparation, and the whole process was underpinned by belief in herself.

Jack

Jack was very successful, having worked his way up to leading a large division of a huge global organisation. Unfortunately, his story of continual achievement and recognition was shattered when he learned that his father had been diagnosed with a terminal illness. Jack and his father were very close, although his career aspirations had meant that they had spent relatively little time together in recent years. Jack continued to work, and helped his mother care for his father when he was able, but he wasn't happy; the situation wasn't right. Against the advice of key people at work, he decided to take an extended leave of absence, knowing that his career would be put on hold and even jeopardised. He went to great lengths to communicate the situation and his reasoning to his team and to ensure that all was in order before he left. He made it clear to his team that he was not to be contacted under any circumstance since he had complete confidence and trust in them.

Jack spent a very rewarding and fulfilling last few months with his father and returned to work with his reputation intact, and respect for him enhanced. He had stuck to his values and beliefs in a manner that had benefited all concerned.

Although he would not have been fully aware of it, Jack had done a great job in dealing with this situation by working through all four mental toughness pillars. He was stressed by having to decide where his priorities lay and he responded in a calm, rational and planned manner. In making the decision to take the leave of absence, he was focusing on the most important thing to him at that time - and he ensured that there would be no work distractions. In handing over total control and responsibility to his team, he demonstrated a belief in himself; he did not need the security of 'feeling indispensable'. Finally, in working out his priorities in life, he was willing to run the risk of jeopardising his career, and the external recognition and rewards that went with it. His motivation was about his intrinsic need to do what was important to him. Here was mental toughness at its best.

So there it is. You are now familiar with the essential elements of mental toughness. Some people are very fortunate in that they appear to be naturally mentally tough. The good news is that it is also possible to develop it. The chapters that follow will take you on your journey.

Chris Andy Scott Emma Studies

Chris (the coach), Andy (the managing director), Scott (the golfer) and Emma (the senior executive) were introduced in Chapter 2. All of them were under pressure and needed to develop their mental toughness. Their situations and mindsets in the context of the four mental toughness pillars are described below.

Chris

Chris was a highly visible coach whose early success started to turn sour as the results went against him. His *focus* turned to things that were going wrong and away from the strengths that he had worked so hard to build. Chris started to question his ability and his waning *belief* led him to start listening to others' views and opinions. The pressure was now causing him *stress* and he was wondering if it was all worthwhile. For the first time, he was concerned about his *motivation* to carry on.

Andy

Andy was a new managing director whose perception that he was constantly under the spotlight and that others were waiting for him to fail was a classic source of self-imposed *stress*. His *focus* was on what others thought of him and this was exacerbated by a lack of *self-belief* reflected in the fact that he was waiting 'to be found out'. Andy's *motivation* was merely to avoid failure.

Scott

Scott was tipped for great things, but his performances in his first year as a professional were not matching others' expectations. His debts were mounting and his *motivation* was becoming more about earning money than it was about enjoying playing the game he loved. Scott's *focus* was on winning and nothing else, and as his performances continued to decline so that elusive win slipped further away and his *stress* began to turn into desperation. His *self-belief* had never been so low.

Emma

Emma spent most of her time *focusing* on being a woman in a male-dominated environment. Her *motivation* was driven by a need to prove herself to her male colleagues. She had *belief* in her ability, but it was manifesting itself in an inflexibility that caused problems in her working relationships. Emma's intense need to be recognised as worthy of her senior position was a major source of the *stress* she experienced.

In a nutshell

- Mental toughness is not the same as being physically and mentally hard, masculine, ruthless, stubborn, suppressing emotions and pushing yourself to extreme limits when it is not sensible to do so.
- Mentally tough performers are often open, fair-minded, caring and decent people who are very good at controlling their thoughts, and acting rationally and in a constructive manner when the pressure is really on.
- Mentally tough performers have high self-awareness and the ability to regulate their thoughts, feelings, emotions and behaviour in a manner that delivers sustained success across a wide range of situations.
- Mental toughness comprises four pillars that form the foundation of sustained high performance:
  - ➢ keeping your head under stress;
  - ➢ staying strong in your self-belief;
  - ➢ making your motivation work for you;
  - ➢ maintaining your focus on the things that matter.
- Mental toughness can be developed.

4 Keeping Your Head Under Stress

After reading this chapter you will know about:

- What stress is and how its affects you
- How to recognise when you are choosing to be stressed
- Strategies and techniques that will help you keep your head under stress

Mentally tough performers are like all of us; they get stressed as well. The key to delivering sustained high performance is that they have developed strategies and techniques that enable them to control stress and keep their heads. This chapter shows how you too can keep your head under stress, but it is important to first establish what stress actually is, and then how pressure and stress are related.

Stress: the dark side of pressure

As the coach was delivering his dressing room team-talk in the bowels of a stadium that eagerly anticipated their grand entrance, my gaze wandered around the faces of the players. These were the last few minutes before their biggest challenge of the year to date – playing against the world champions in front of a full house. Their faces spoke a thousand words. It was easy to pick out those who were loving every single moment of this pressure-cooker environment. The desire and intense focus was etched in their eyes; this was what the long hours and hard work devoted to training was all about. They were just about to enter an arena they craved and existed for. Some other faces portrayed a very different experience. Their frightened eyes, and the tension and paleness in their faces, reflected the torture of their nerve-racked bodies and the fear of failure on such an enormous stage. I had the impression that their souls had never been so severely tested before.

The scene I was witnessing represented the two 'faces' of pressure shown in Figure 4.1 – at its best it exhilarates and energises; at its worst it crushes and drains performers. The negative side of pressure is otherwise known as stress, that often unpleasant and debilitating consequence of not coping with pressure.

I have witnessed the two faces of pressure in business too. Faced with impossible targets in the run-up to the flotation of an organisation, senior figures were working ridiculous hours with sleepless nights in between. These people were certainly not thriving on the pressure! And imagine the stress experienced by the senior leadership team of a manufacturing company whose early-year forecast of a healthy profit turned very quickly into a substantial loss and closure of one of their plants, simply as a result of successive substantial and uncontrollable hikes in energy prices. Stress was also a major factor for employees in a large organisation that experienced a year-long period of uncertainty surrounding a much publicised takeover. The uncertainty, together with a lack of control, were the key ingredients for widespread stress.

Figure 4.1 The two faces of pressure.

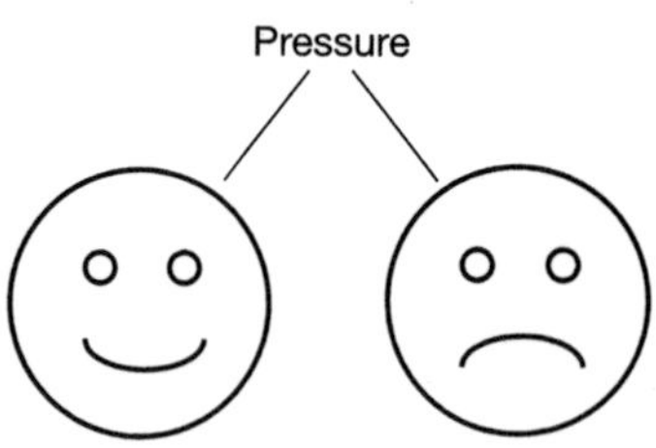

Stress is not always caused by the type of major events described above. It can simply be the result of the daily grind, hassles and sometimes monotony of work getting on top of you. Or maybe it is a result of the incessant performance demands wearing you down. Often in such situations, stress is the result of self-perpetuating distorted perceptions that you are not in control, an important area that is addressed later in this chapter.

Stress can take two forms; acute and chronic.

Acute stress

Acute stress is characterised by bouts of stress interspersed with periods of little or no stress. You may find yourself relatively stressed during the working day, but if the stress then subsides significantly when you are away from the performing environment, then you are experiencing acute stress. Human beings are pretty well equipped to deal with acute stress and can cope with it for prolonged periods, although it is important to build in rest periods to wind down and replenish vital energy stores.

Chronic Stress

Chronic stress is where the bouts of stress run into one another. You get home from work and are unable to switch off from the things that are frustrating you. You may even lie awake at night re-running the events of the day and worrying about the day to follow. This form of stress is not good for you if it occurs over prolonged periods. Your immune system starts to wear down and you become susceptible to infections and illnesses. If it has just occurred to you that you may have been suffering from what appears to be chronic stress over the last few weeks, you may be starting to worry. Don't panic! It takes considerably longer for this form of stress to cause serious health problems, but people with chronic stress should certainly take action sooner rather than later.

Over to Adrian . . .

I *always* swam faster in races than in training. I needed to have the pressure of racing rivals to perform at my best. The harder thing to manage was the daily grind of training. I would often get so tired that I couldn't lift my arms, and would walk through the door after morning training and sleep until lunchtime. This kind of fatigue would lead to me arguing with the people closest to me which was definitely a source of considerable stress. Also, I would occasionally worry that I was not training hard enough, or whether I was doing the right thing. This was a sign that the pressure was getting to me and turning into stress.

So far, I have depicted stress as the dark side of pressure. This needs to be qualified. Some (acute) stress is good; indeed, throughout the whole of human existence on earth it has served the very important function of alerting and preparing you for potential danger. And in today's fast-moving world, it can help to focus you on key priorities and to mobilise the resources required to perform. However, excessive levels of stress act as a distracter and result in impaired performance. The ability to control stress to manageable proportions is therefore very important and a core pillar of mental toughness.

What do you do with your stress?

The key to being able to control your stress is awareness. People are often stressed without fully realising it. Have you ever taken a holiday after a prolonged busy period at work and been really puzzled why you feel particularly tired, or have unexplained aches and pains, or maybe niggling headaches or a cold? The probability is that you have been experiencing some stress and have been coping with it because you have to, and it's never been severe enough to cause you any significant problems. That is what tends to happen with stress – you have it, but aren't always aware of it because you are able to keep going. But it will get you at some point. Taking time out to relax provides it with a perfect opportunity – you lower your defences and in it comes!

Recognising what you do with your stress and what it does to you is therefore pretty important. Have a look at the list of stress categories below. Do you recognise yourself in any of them?

- **Stress hoarder** – you keep your stress to yourself so that others are often unaware of it. You appear calm and in control to the outside world, but this merely hides an inner turmoil.
- **Stress delegator** – you knowingly pass your stress on to other people to deal with. You see lots of other people under stress when you feel fine.
- **Stress carrier** – you may not experience too much stress yourself, but unwittingly cause lots for other people. You notice people turn on their heels as they catch sight of you and disappear hotfoot in the opposite direction.
- **Stress protector** – you protect other people from stress by taking it on board yourself. You see yourself as a warrior who rescues people from their stress.
- **Stress avoider** – you do not put yourself in situations that are likely to cause stress. You lead a safe, unstimulating, comfortable existence.

- **Stress sponge** – you feel that you can cope with any amount of stress. You put yourself in as many difficult and challenging situations as possible.
- **Stress rationaliser** – you accept stress as part of life. You view it as something you must learn to cope with and are relatively uncomplaining and 'just get on with things' during times of stress.
- **Stress buster** – you view life as too short to have to bother about stress and confront issues that cause it head-on in an effort to sort them out.
- **Stress denier** – you refuse to accept you are under stress, despite feedback to the contrary. You consider it to be a sign of weakness to admit that you are stressed.
- **Stress magnet** – you seem to be constantly stressed. You wonder why you always feel out of sorts.

Over to Adrian . . .

Over the years in sport and business, I have met almost every stress category! Some people seem to manage, and even succeed with their own method of coping. Mostly they can't sustain it though. I believe I fall into the 'rationaliser' category, and I'm sure it has come from experiences with my parents as I mentioned earlier, as well as coming through a huge personal disappointment such as the 1984 Olympics. I think that I accept *pressure* as part of my life. I also accept responsibility for choosing the life I am leading. I guess that I have found strategies to cope that help me before getting *too* stressed. Some are mental, and some are physical (planned) – for example, I have not worked a weekend for many years, and I always take my full holiday allowance. I build in time for 'restoration'.

Tackling and controlling stress levels to manageable proportions can present an enormous challenge and often requires a structured approach at three levels:

1 identifying the sources of pressure that can result in stress;

2 recognising when you are stressed;

3 developing suitable coping strategies and techniques.

The model described in the following sections has proved particularly useful in facilitating both business and sport performers' development in these three areas.

Stress: what is it and what are its effects?

The huge literature on stress and how to cope with it is full of different perspectives, sometimes conflicting definitions and hence different approaches to how to treat it. This reflects an area that has attracted a considerable amount of interest due to its seemingly increasing prevalence and impact in modern society, but it also reflects a topic that is complex and difficult to get to grips with. 'Stress' is a term that is used in everyday life to cover a multitude of situations and responses. In the medical profession, for example, general practitioners tend to use stress as a catch all diagnosis of numerous ailments that have no apparent physical explanation. In such circumstances, it is relatively easy to find perplexed employers without key people who present them with sick notes declaring themselves unfit for work in the absence of any obvious signs of ill health.

Some clarity around stress and its effects is therefore crucial before developing strategies for coping with it. The model shown in Figure 4.2 is the culmination of my own research together with my efforts to make sense of the more meaningful trends in thinking in the scientific literature. It represents a simple and very practical way of viewing stress and its effects, leading to how to cope with it. The key components of the model, described in the following sections, are essentially the sources of pressure that may lead to stress, the way you are in terms of your predispositions to experience and deal with pressure, how you appraise or think about pressure and how this may result in stress, and finally, how stress affects you.

Figure 4.2 The stress process.

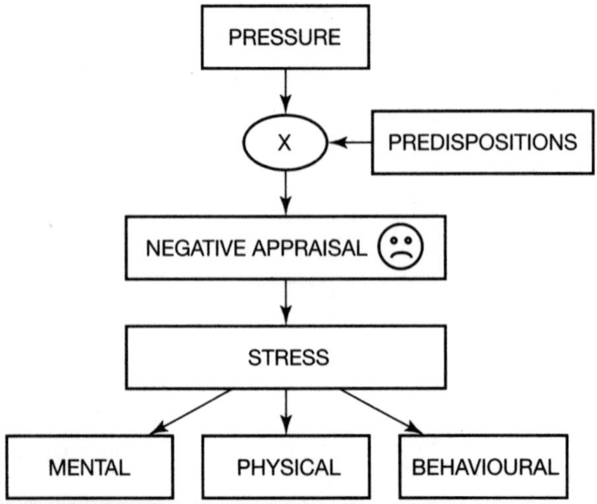

Pressure: what gets to you?

I described in Chapter 2 how pressure can originate from two sources – external and internal. The pressure referred to here is that which is imposed on you from the external environment. In addition to the internal-external distinction, pressure can also be thought of as being either 'unconscious' or 'conscious'. Gravity is a rather extreme example of unconscious pressure, but serves as an appropriate illustration because it is common to everyone. Gravity is essentially a constant source of pressure that is pulling you towards the ground. It is only a complex musculoskeletal system that allows you to cope with this pressure, otherwise you would be lying in a heap on the floor! Indeed, this system is so effective that you are rarely conscious of gravity at all. Only when you put the system under too much strain – following an excessive intake of alcohol, for example – are you alerted to this source of pressure.

Your unconscious sources of pressure might be things that you take for granted, such as regularly driving to the office in heavy traffic, or perhaps always ensuring you get home at a reasonable time to spend some quality time with your loved ones in order to satisfy their and your needs. Unconscious pressures are potentially dangerous, because you don't bring them to your conscious attention and thus you do nothing to alleviate them. Over time, these pressures slowly eat away at and deplete valuable energy and focus resources that are core to your daily performance. Making yourself conscious of these pressures and their impact and then doing something about them is clearly very important. In the same way that your musculoskeletal system requires regular rest to maximise its effectiveness, so too does your mind.

Try to identify some things that you take for granted (you may need someone else's help with this), such as the journey to and from work, and think about how they might be linked to any stress you experience. You may surprise yourself!

Now consider the pressures that you are conscious of, perhaps in the form of those daily demands of providing 'numbers updates' to challenging colleagues at meetings or hitting those looming deadlines. Then there are the more major sources of pressure such as delivering important presentations, negotiating those crucial deals or competing for a particularly big piece of business. These are the sources of pressure that you are acutely aware of and demand your focus. They may keep you awake at night, but at least you are conscious of them and thus in a position to deal with them in a constructive manner. What are the sources of pressure that you are particularly conscious of?

Over to Adrian . . .

The conscious sources of pressure for me as a swimmer were the obvious ones like competing and putting in quality training sessions day-in-day-out. I was always really aware of these demands.

Possible unconscious sources of pressure from my swimming days probably included things like getting early nights. I always made myself get to bed before 10pm if I could, because it wasn't enough just to arrive at the following morning training sessions at 5.30am, but to arrive in a state to be able to physically perform. Early nights meant a number of decisions and choices to be taken.

Something else, which I almost took for granted when I became the World Number One, was the constant scrutiny of the swimming world at large. It wasn't necessarily the press attention, but just people connected to the sport who always seemed to be 'interested' in me and my life...!

Now I look back on it, these were probably bigger factors in my life than I realised at the time.

Predispositions: are you your own worst enemy?

Take a few moments to reflect on how you normally respond to pressure. Does it tend to debilitate or aid your performance? This element of the model essentially deals with your own propensity to impose pressure on yourself which, in turn, may turn into stress. Consider the examples of delivering an important presentation or being interviewed for a top position. If these are not particularly relevant to you, then use a source of pressure that you identified in the previous section as a frame of reference. The way you respond in these situations will be the function of the interaction of a number of factors and predispositions that you take with you into them. Particularly significant ones are described below.

Beliefs and attitudes

These essentially relate to how you think and feel about the sources of pressure. You may enjoy and look forward to presenting or being interviewed because you are very good at it, or because of the great pleasure you get from the excitement of the adrenaline rush. Or you may view it as a necessary part of what you do so that you should just accept and get on with it. On the other hand, delivering an important presentation or being interviewed may be something you dread. This could be because you perceive yourself to be unable to perform at your best, or perhaps because you do not enjoy, and are debilitated by, the nerves you experience beforehand.

Over to Adrian . . .

As I mentioned earlier, I think that my perspective on life changed quite a lot after my defeat at the 1984 Olympics. I realised that by swimming, I was just enjoying doing something that I had found a talent for, and that I was in a very fortunate position to be continuing to be doing it through to my mid-to-late 20s. It also dawned on me that winning or losing swimming races didn't have much impact on the world at large, and so I should relax and enjoy the thrill of racing. In essence I stopped being afraid of losing.

Past experiences

These fall into two categories – general and specific.

General experiences refer to how you feel about your previous important presentations or major interviews. This will be based on how you dealt with the nerves, any feedback you received and your own perceptions of how you performed. In this way, past general experiences will, to some extent, determine how you feel about upcoming presentations or interviews.

Specific experiences refer to the similarities between upcoming situations and past experiences. For example, if you have presented to this same audience on a previous occasion, then how you feel about the upcoming presentation will inevitably be strongly related to how it went with the same audience in the past. In the same way, sport performers often associate some venues with good or poor performances in the past, and this will influence their thoughts and feelings before future performances at the same venues.

Personality

Research shows that the personality that is formed in your early years remains relatively unchanged throughout your life. This doesn't mean that you have to think or behave in the same way forever – indeed, the whole premise of developing mental toughness is based on the principle of being able to moderate thoughts and behaviour – but it does mean that you are hard-wired to respond in certain ways across different situations. In fact, highly pressured situations are often the stimulus for your personality traits to come to the fore. There are many different facets of personality which are beyond the scope of this chapter, but there are three dimensions that are particularly important in how you respond to pressure.

- **Trait anxiety** – this simply reflects the level of proneness to become anxious across a variety of situations. High trait anxiety people are likely to become anxious in most situations involving any pressure.
- **Optimism-pessimism** – this dimension of personality speaks for itself. Optimists are likely to be more positive about coping with and performing well under pressure than pessimists. Consequently, pessimists are more prone to experience stress than optimists.
- **Perfectionism** – for people high on perfectionism, the need to do things perfectly adds even more pressure, making them more prone to experience stress than people low on perfectionism.

Over to Adrian . . .

More often than not it is in my nature is to be optimistic. I do tend to see the best in a situation or person – until proved differently. At the heart of that thinking is the belief that life is a gift, and that grumbling or whining just gets in the way of making the most of the joy of life. Consequently, whenever faced with pressure I do ask myself 'what's the worst that can happen?' Due to my optimism, I am sure that I always come back with the right answer for me at the time, and that is usually something like . . . 'well, it could all go pear-shaped, but will I lose my life? No? Ok then, let's have a go . . . ' I am sure that I choose to opt in or out of situations as well, depending on my abilities to cope. I'm not a stress junkie, I know when to back off!

Think about predispositions you are aware of that are significant influences in determining how you respond to pressured situations. In particular, think about how they influence how you respond to each of the specific pressure sources you identified in the previous section.

Appraisal: do you choose to be stressed?

The doctor is examining the child's growth. What image does this statement create in your mind – a doctor measuring a child's height or examining a cancerous growth? Isn't it amazing that such a neutral statement can conjure up such wildly differing images? The key to the whole stress response is that you had a choice over which image you generated – you chose to apply either a positive perspective in terms of height, or a negative perspective in imaging a child with cancer. This leads to the crucial factor about stress – most of it is self-imposed! How you think about or appraise pressure determines whether you are stressed by it. The basic choice you have is between viewing the pressure as either positive in terms of providing an opportunity, or negative in that it poses a threat. A positive appraisal will normally result in feelings such as exhilaration and excitement; a negative appraisal usually results in stress and feeling anxious.

The problem is that you are not always in complete control of your choice to be stressed or not. Your predisposition to pressure and stress means that you have biases in your perception and interpretation of situations. For example, high trait anxiety people have a tendency to naturally view most pressure as involving some threat. Pessimists are likely to approach pressure situations anticipating that they will be unable to cope and will underperform, a biased appraisal that inevitably causes stress. And put pessimism together with high perfectionism and you have someone who must perform perfectly, but won't! Imagine the stress experienced by a person with this appraisal.

The realisation that you have a choice about how you think about and appraise pressure is the first crucial aspect of controlling stress. The second is recognising your predisposition to experience stress and the impact that has on how you view and approach it. Before moving on to the next section, reflect on your sources of pressure and the predispositions that influence how you respond to each. What are the resulting appraisals that you typically arrive at in those situations and circumstances?

Response: how does stress affect you?

Think back to your most recent memory of being stressed. It may be that you were having a negative response to the pressure of that really important presentation or that big interview or assessment centre. What were you thinking, how was your body responding, and how were you behaving? Although the stress response is specific to individuals, it can be broken down into three major types of symptom that are common to everyone:

- **Mental** – including things like doubt, worry, poor memory recall, frustration, confusion and panic.
- **Physical** – including muscle tension, pounding heart, sickness, butterflies and sweaty palms.
- **Behavioural** – including fidgeting, pacing, becoming quiet and withdrawn or maybe loud and outgoing, being short-tempered, drinking excessive amounts of caffeine and alcohol, and disturbed sleep.

Do you recognise any of these symptoms in yourself? They are by no means exhaustive and there will be many others that are specific to you and particular stressful situations. The key to dealing with symptoms of stress is recognising when you are experiencing them and that it's stress that's actually causing them. This last point is particularly important when making assumptions about other people who *look* stressed. For example, you may have a colleague or team member who always seems to be running around like the proverbial headless chicken, always short of time and having too much to do. Far from being stressed, this person may be thriving on the pressure and may only get stressed when there isn't enough to do and boredom sets in. Being aware of 'normal' responses and subtle changes in behaviour is the key to supporting other people under stress. For example, there is something awry with a golfer who normally takes two practice swings before playing every iron shot, but takes one or three before a particular shot. The key point is to look for the more subtle changes in others' behaviour as a sign of potential stress.

Over to Adrian . . .

Breaking down the stress response into mental, physical and behavioural components helps me to better understand how stress affected me during my early swimming years. Whilst still living at home with my parents, I found some of the winter training extremely hard to cope with and not just due to the physical pain. Often, when returning home extremely frustrated and angry (mental) after a particularly bad session, my mother would innocently ask how it had gone. I sometimes stormed off up to my room, with a monosyllabic grunt if I was in a good mood, or shouting and slamming doors if I wasn't . . . (behavioural).

During competition, these symptoms would be heightened. I would sometimes have a negative voice in my head that was louder than the positive one (mental). The little guy with the 'you can do it' chant of encouragement was often drowned out by a louder and more aggressive voice telling me that 'you can't possibly'. Before an important race I would find myself becoming quite tense in the shoulders and back (physical). Luckily we had physiotherapists travelling with the team! When it got to the last half an hour before the race you could spot some of the more stressed competitors – usually by their fidgety behaviour. Some would just pace back and forth in the changing rooms, whilst others would sit in a corner with a towel over their head.

Work on identifying subtle changes in your own thoughts, feelings and behaviour when you are stressed. Someone who knows you well can help you with pinpointing subtle behavioural changes and when they occur. In particular, think about the symptoms you experience in response to the specific stress sources you experience. This will alert you to when you are becoming stressed and the need to take action to control it.

You have hopefully given careful consideration to the questions posed throughout this section and have generated some valuable reflections on key aspects of what causes you stress and how you respond to it. This level of awareness and understanding is fundamental to enabling you to develop strategies and techniques for controlling stress and its effects. Spend a few minutes capturing your reflections and conclusions in Time-Out 4.1 below before moving on to the next section.

Time-Out 4.1

Stress and how it affects you

Pressure: what gets to you?

- What are the pressures you take for granted and how might they be linked to any stress you experience? (You may need someone else's help with this.)
- What are the pressures you are particularly conscious of and how are they linked to any stress you experience?

Predispositions: are you your own worst enemy?

- What are the predispositions (personality, past experiences, attitudes, beliefs, values, etc) you are aware of that are significant influences in determining how you respond to pressure?
- How do these predispositions influence how you respond to the various pressures you identified in the previous section?

Appraisal: do you choose to be stressed?

- Reflecting back on your sources of pressure and the predispositions that influence how you respond, what are the appraisals that you typically arrive at in those situations and circumstances?
- How are these appraisals linked to any stress you experience?

Response: how does stress affect you?

- What are the mental, physical and behavioural symptoms you are aware of when you are stressed?
- What are the subtle changes in your thoughts, feelings and behaviours when you are stressed? (Someone who knows you well can help you pinpoint subtle behavioural changes and when they occur.)

Stress: how to control it and keep your head

In the same way that you almost always have a choice over whether to be stressed or not, so you also have a choice over how to cope when you *are* stressed. There are essentially three types of strategy for controlling stress, as shown in Figure 4.3: controlling the effects of stress or *symptom-focused strategies*; challenging the thinking that causes you stress or *appraisal-focused strategies*; and tackling the situations and circumstances that cause you stress or *situation-focused strategies*.

Figure 4.3 Stress and coping strategies.

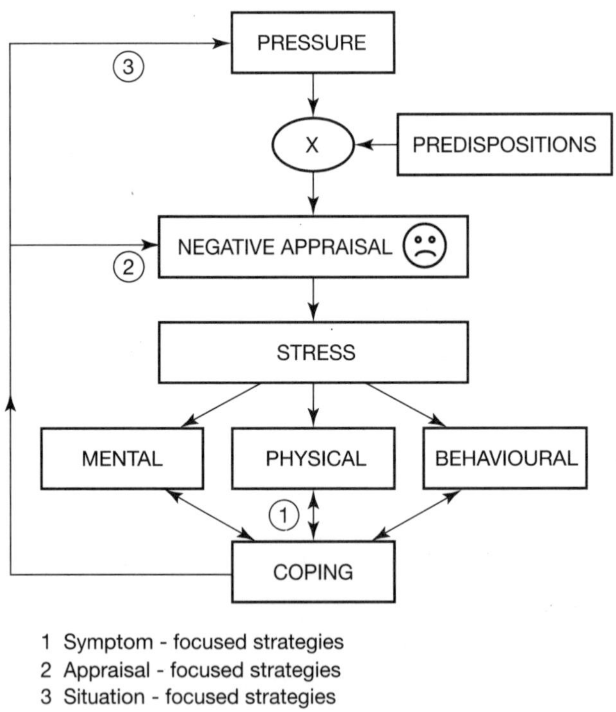

Controlling the effects of stress: symptom-focused strategies

Symptom-focused strategies target the stress symptoms themselves and attempt to control them to manageable proportions. As emphasised in the previous section, recognising the symptoms that you experience when you are stressed and being aware of when you are experiencing them is crucial. Breaking the symptoms down into mental, physical and behavioural components is helpful in leading you to an appropriate means of controlling them.

Controlling mental symptoms

Mental symptoms, often in the form of things like doubt, worry, frustration and anger, are most effectively controlled by mental relaxation. Mental relaxation can be broken down into two broad areas. Firstly, relaxation can be in the form of enjoyable activities that serve to distract you from the pressure of performing. Activities commonly cited as helping to take people's mind off things include exercise, listening to music, reading, walking the dog, gardening and the like. Secondly, mental relaxation can be of a more formal nature with the main objective being to provide your mind and body with rest.

A common form of mental relaxation is **meditation**, which typically comprises concentrating on breathing and using a mantra or keyword spoken silently on each exhalation. This technique is based on the principle of distracting you from negative thoughts and focusing you instead on the mantra or keyword as a means of clearing and calming your mind. I have used meditative relaxation with both business and sport performers who have experienced intense mental symptoms when under stress. They have typically learned three forms of relaxation: deep, intermediate and quick forms (scripts for all three forms of meditative relaxation are provided in Appendix A).

1. The **deep** form of meditative relaxation, typically lasting between 15–20 minutes, is generally practised sitting or lying down and with your eyes shut. You then progress through various stages as follows:
   - focusing on your breathing;
   - focusing on saying 'one' silently to yourself on each breath out.
   - counting down from 10 to 1 on each successive breath out;

- focusing on saying 'one' to yourself;
- counting up from 1 to 7 on each breath in;
- opening your eyes.

2 The **intermediate** form of meditative relaxation is essentially a shortened version of the deep form and is practised over approximately 5–6 minutes. It can be used as a means of composing yourself in those final hours or minutes in the run-up to that important event.

3. The **quick** form of meditative relaxation can be performed over a few seconds as a means of re-focusing or calming your mind in those crucial moments during performance. This simply involves focusing on the mantra or keyword over three or four breaths out. Executives I have worked with use this quick form of relaxation to compose themselves before important presentations or maybe to manage any anger, frustration or other negative emotions when it is important that they are kept under tight control.

Over to Adrian . . .

Basic breathing exercises were some of the most-used forms of relaxation for me, particularly in the ready room before a big final. If the race itself wasn't stressful enough, we had to report to a room with our fellow finalists for half an hour before the race. Sitting there with only your own mind for company could sometimes get a little testing. I used to count and control my breathing, taking in deeper and longer breaths. This was mainly a calming technique, a by-product being that it stopped my adrenalin from kicking in too early.

Another effective technique for dealing with mental symptoms of stress is **imagery-based relaxation**. The principles underlying the effectiveness of imagery-based relaxation are similar to those of meditative relaxation – it simply acts as a means of distracting you from your negative mental symptoms and focusing you instead on thoughts that calm your mind. Focusing for a few minutes or even seconds on an image of something or somewhere you find very relaxing, such as lying on a beach, soaking in a warm bath, or perhaps walking though beautiful countryside, will help to compose your troubled mind (see Appendix B for a sample imagery-based relaxation script and suggestions for developing your own).

Over to Adrian . . .

Because I used to travel far and wide to compete, I often would find myself imagining being back at home, walking on a hillside in the Yorkshire Dales. Big, wide open spaces with lots of air to breathe. A real contrast to some of the pokey rooms I would be sitting in down in the bowels of a swimming pool, waiting to walk out for an Olympic final! This was one of my main forms of relaxation - just to spend a little time daydreaming and changing my mental focus.

You will also be able to develop your own ways of controlling the content of your conscious mind. As long as you adhere to the key principles involved in first of all recognising that the thoughts filling your conscious mind are unhelpful, and then taking a few minutes or seconds to replace them with more positive thoughts, experiment and find what works for you.

Controlling physical symptoms

Physical symptoms are those bodily reactions that can be quite unpleasant; the headache, those jelly legs, the sometimes uncomfortable muscle tension, the pounding heart, that feeling of sickness, the butterflies or perhaps an empty feeling in the pit of your stomach, the sweaty palms, the voice tremor and sometimes uncontrollable muscles in your face that betray the nerves, anger or frustration you are trying so desperately to hide.

An effective technique for dealing with the physical symptoms of stress is **progressive muscular relaxation** (PMR). As with meditative relaxation, PMR can be used to generate a deeply relaxed state if performed over 15–20 minutes, or a few second version will help to relax or loosen up certain muscle groups as required. PMR generally involves tensing and relaxing various muscle groups and progressing through the body in a structured manner. As with meditation, the length of the PMR can be customised to meet specific needs. The ultimate goal for performers is to derive benefit from it within a few seconds. For example, you may have seen tennis players tensing and relaxing the muscles in their forearms in between rallies – this is to quickly get rid of any unwanted tension that will impair their 'feel' of the ball on the racket. Again, this technique is easily applicable and transferable to business performers who want to release any unwanted physical tension before a presentation or during an important meeting (see Appendix C for a PMR script).

Over to Adrian . . .

I would use PMR mainly in the time I had between prelims and finals. At the major events, we would race the prelims in the morning and then have four or five hours' rest before racing the final in the evening. Having swum a fast and exacting race to qualify for the final, I sometimes found myself lying on my bed thinking about the evening race and getting quite tense.

Another effective way of dealing with the physical symptoms of stress is **abdominal breathing**. Your breathing reflects the level of tension you carry in your body. When you are tense, your breathing usually becomes shallow and rapid, involving the upper chest area only. When you are relaxed, you breathe more fully and deeply, and from your abdomen. Learning to breathe in this way can help you alleviate the physical symptoms of stress, and even result in a relaxed state when you become proficient at it. Appendix D shows you how to reduce tension by breathing from the abdomen.

Controlling behavioural symptoms

Behavioural symptoms of stress are those that are observable: nervous fidgeting or pacing, becoming quiet and withdrawn or maybe loud and outgoing, drinking excessive amounts of caffeine and alcohol, being irritable, and many more that are too numerous to mention here. In keeping with the basic theme for this entire chapter, the key is to develop awareness and in this case to recognise how your behaviour changes when you are stressed. Your behavioural changes need not be dramatic, but instead quite subtle, as described earlier in this chapter. Work through your behavioural changes and identify those which are unhelpful during different phases of your performance cycle. For example, if you drink an excessive amount of caffeine-laced coffee during periods of stress and this exacerbates your sleeping problem, then there is a pretty easy solution to this particular symptom!

Over to Adrian . . .

Looking back on it, I had several approaches to dealing with my stress symptoms. I would read a book, do crosswords or listen to music – all internal things to take my mind away and be in a different place. I also moved away from nervous people. I would never be around teammates or coaches who couldn't cope.

I could always tell when my coach was really nervous before a race, because when we had the final talk before I went to report to the ready room, his behaviour gave it away. He used to screw his programme up and started talking more quickly. So in the end I used to tell him that I would see him an hour and a half beforehand, and that would be the only time I would see him.

In swimming the hardest time before the race is the half hour leading up to it. That's when it becomes quite gladiatorial as you're with your seven opponents in the room waiting. Your breathing becomes quicker and muscles start tensing. So I learned ways to deal with that – breathing exercises, basic meditative and muscular relaxation techniques, as I mentioned above.

One useful tool to help me cope with the competition stress came from a conversation with a sport psychologist. I was talking about how the negative voice in my head sometimes appeared to be louder than the more positive one. To get over this I visualised the bigger voice as being the diminished person and gave the small, more positive guy a megaphone!

Symptom-focused strategies for controlling stress can be very effective and you should devote time and effort to practising and experimenting with the techniques described above. They will prove invaluable in those moments and minutes when stress threatens to overpower you and you need to regain your composure. However, controlling symptoms is only really effective in the short term because you never actually tackle the source of stress and so the symptoms keep returning. The remaining strategies focus, therefore, on techniques that are effective on a longer-term basis.

→ Challenging the thinking that causes you stress: appraisal-focused strategies

I will not pretend that changing negative appraisal and thinking into positive thinking is easy. And for some people who have natural tendencies or predispositions to look on the dark side, it can be a major challenge. The starting point is the realisation and acceptance that you have a choice about the way you think, and that you can actually alter your mode of thinking. Awareness, once again, underpins any change you wish to make. Have a look through the typical negative thought patterns below and note those that you engage in when under pressure:

- **Catastrophising** – thinking the worst has happened, or may or will happen: 'I'm not properly prepared for the presentation tomorrow – it will be a disaster.'
- **Over-generalising** – applying your own thoughts, feelings and attitudes across all people and situations: 'This lot always ask me awkward questions during my presentation.'
- **Discounting the positive** – focusing on the negative aspects of your performance and ignoring the positive: 'Nothing went right.'
- **Mind reading** – making assumptions about what others are thinking and with negative repercussions for yourself: 'The boss looks bored. He's not interested in what I'm saying.'
- **Negative predictions** – looking into the future and predicting a negative outcome: 'I'll never be ready for the presentation.'
- **Black and white thinking** – viewing the world in an either/or context, with little scope for the grey areas: 'The boss was wrong to ask me that question.'
- **Take things personally** – viewing failures or negative feedback as a reflection of your own shortcomings: 'They said my presentation could have focused more on the vision than the strategy. I'm useless.'

Are any of them familiar? I would be surprised if you did not engage in at least one of these thought patterns, because most people do! But they only serve to provoke and exacerbate the stress you experience and therefore need to be countered. Spend a few minutes working through Time-Out 4.2 below to identify any negative thought patterns *you* engage in and how they are linked to stress.

Time-Out 4.2

Do you engage in negative thought patterns?

- Do you engage in any of the following negative thought patterns: catastrophising, over-generalising, discounting the positive, mind reading, negative predictions, black and white thinking, taking things personally?
- How are they linked to any stress you experience?

Over to Adrian . . .

For me, the techniques and strategies I described using in the previous section are the most basic ways of coping with stress, mainly at the symptom level. I still use these techniques today, but the most used method for me became the way I would re-appraise the situation. It was always a good thing to head those symptoms off at the pass if I could. So, mostly, I was trying to re-assess the way I was looking at the situation.

There are several ways of changing or at least modifying your appraisal of pressured situations that enable you to control stress to manageable levels. These are described in the following sections

Taking an 'adult' perspective

One approach that I have found particularly useful in helping performers (and myself!) deal more effectively with pressure is Transactional Analysis.[15] It has proved to be really beneficial in helping people understand the origins of their negative appraisals so that they are better placed to deal with them. The key principle underlying Transactional Analysis is that you are three people in one – a Child, a Parent and an Adult. Sometimes you behave, think and feel as the little child you once were, sometimes in a parental way copied from what you heard and saw in your parents (or parental substitutes), and sometimes as an Adult who analyses, predicts and makes decisions on the basis of objectively-processed data. You assume the perspective of one or another of these people at any given time and can change from one to another in a moment. And it can be very noticeable; your vocabulary, gestures and voice tone are all likely to alter.

Imagine that you are driving your car and approaching a set of traffic lights. As you reach the lights they turn to red so that you find yourself at the front of a queue of three or four cars that are going straight ahead. Another car draws up alongside you in the adjacent and previously unoccupied lane that is for turning off to the right, but you suspect that

[15] The concept of Transactional Analysis was developed by Dr Eric Berne who published the book *Games People Play: The Psychology of Human Relationships*, in 1964. There are many facets to Transactional Analysis that are too broad and numerous to dwell on in this book. This insight draws on selected facets that are particularly pertinent to understanding stress and how to deal with it.

the driver intends to go straight ahead as well. You think to yourself 'Want to race, do you? Come on then', and then slam the accelerator to the floor as the lights change from amber to green. You win the 'race' and the other car is forced to pull in behind you. This is the Child in you, reflected by the immaturity of placing yourself and others at risk for the sake of a 'game', as you would have done when you were a small child.

Far from falling behind and conceding defeat, the driver stays close on your tail looking for any opportunity to overtake. Your thoughts turn to 'the ridiculous driving of the guy behind' and 'he shouldn't be allowed on the road'. You become intent on showing him how to drive and slow down to the legal speed limit, forcing the car behind to follow suit. This is the Parent in you, in which you are in the same state of mind as one of your parents (or parental substitute) used to be, and you respond as s/he would with the same postures, gestures, vocabulary, feelings, etc. You can now see that the driver behind is getting extremely irritated and you start to wonder why overtaking you is so important to him. You think to yourself, 'perhaps he's late for a meeting, or perhaps he's been called home because of some emergency situation' and you pull over to allow the car to make rapid progress on its journey. This is the Adult in you which allows you to make an objective appraisal of the situation and respond in a non-prejudicial manner.

Replaying early experiences

What underpins this process? Research[16] has shown that the brain acts like a tape recorder, so that whilst we may 'forget' our early childhood experiences, recordings of them remain within the brain locked together with the associated feelings. These recorded experiences and associated feelings are available for replay today as vividly as when they actually happened so that events in the present can replicate an old experience and cause the same response.

The Child

The Child in you is filled with desire and motivation. It is often the most delightful part of yourself when it is free to be spontaneous, inventive, creative, fun-loving and carefree. The Child can also be a problem when it manifests in immature, over-competitive, over-emotional, rebellious, aggressive and selfish thoughts and behaviours. Language used in internal dialogue and external communication whilst in the Child state will

---

[16] Wilder Penfield. Memory Mechanisms, *AMA Archives of Neurology and Psychiatry*, 67, 178–198, 1952.

include things like 'I want', 'I need', 'I like', 'I don't like', 'I'm helpless', 'It's her fault not mine', 'If he can so can I', 'I feel guilty', 'I'm scared', and 'If I fail here I'm in real trouble'.

The Parent

The Parent in you reflects traditions and values and a way of life that was taught and demonstrated to you by your parents (or parental substitutes) at a very young age. Behaviour is copied from others, together with associated beliefs, values and opinions. It decides, without reasoning, how to react to situations, what is good or bad, and how people should live. The Parent has a nurturing and caring side and a set of rules and boundaries that are designed to keep people safe. On the other hand, the Parent can be overbearing and can smother with concern, denying people the opportunity to develop their own skills. Language used in internal dialogue and external communication whilst in the Parent state will include things like 'right', 'wrong', 'good', 'bad', 'never', 'ought', 'must', 'should', 'what will people say?' and 'why didn't I …'.

The Adult

A person in the Adult state appears thoughtful, rational and in the here and now. The Adult serves the important function of controlling the Child's impulses and the Parent's moralistic demands by ensuring that information is gathered to make a rational decision. Language used in internal dialogue and external communication whilst in the Adult state will include things like 'what's the evidence?', 'what do you think?', 'what are the options?', 'what are the choices?', 'I don't want to make a rash decision here' and 'I don't have enough information to go on'.

Effects in time of pressure

Since Transactional Analysis emphasises the importance of early events and experiences, and how you were as a child and how your parents (or parental substitutes) were with you, the likelihood of assuming the Child or Parent part of you in given situations is quite prominent. This can have a big impact on how you appraise pressured situations. Consider how you think and react under a specific source of pressure, say in your appraisal of a performance failure or setback. In the Child state, you might think things like, 'I feel really bad about failing', 'I'm scared what will happen if I mess up again', 'I don't know what to do about it', 'if only I'd listened to the advice'. Such thoughts are likely to culminate in stress in the form of guilt, fear, helplessness and/or regret. In the Parent state, you might think things like 'I must never do that again', 'I should have done it that way', 'I've let everyone down', 'what will people think of me?'. These thoughts are likely to result in stress due to remorse, failure to adhere to 'norms', worry about others' perceptions and/or distorted value-judgements.

The Child and the Parent parts of you are, therefore, potential enemies in times of pressure. It is important that you are able to recognise the state you have adopted and to step out of it so that you can weigh up the evidence to support or refute your negative thoughts. This is only possible in the Adult state in which you might think things like 'are these thoughts rational?', 'is there another way of looking at it?', 'how can I take some learning from this?', 'what went well and how would I do things differently next time?'. This way of thinking does not reflect denial – the important thing is to recognise the failure, but to then deal with it in a way that allows you to move forward constructively.

Using the Adult to deal with pressure

Now think about a pressured event or set of circumstances that will occur in the future, say in the form of performance goals that have been set for you. The Child in you is likely to think about them in a manner that distracts you from your purpose and at the same time induces stress – 'I want to do better than everyone else', 'why are their targets lower than mine?', 'I'm afraid of the consequences if I fail', 'I'll never do it'. Stress will be created by the Parent in the form of thoughts like 'I must achieve them', 'I mustn't let them down', 'I can't ask for help – that's a sign of weakness'. The Adult in you will take a different perspective – 'let's plan how I can achieve them', 'what are the various ways in which I might achieve them?', 'what support do I require?', 'this is really stretching, but this is why I'm here'.

The Adult in you is clearly crucial in enabling you to deal constructively with pressure. It controls the Parent and Child parts of you so that you are able to appraise the information at your disposal in a logical and rational manner. This does not mean that you should do away with the Parent and Child altogether. They can play a very important role under pressure, with the Parent being aware of potential danger and the Child enabling you to derive some fun and see the lighter side of highly pressured situations. The goal is the strengthening and anticipation of the Adult so that you slow down and assess your thoughts, recognising that you actually have a free choice about how to respond. Awareness, as with any area of self-development, is the starting point. With this aim in mind, record your own typical Parent, Adult and Child responses to pressure in Time-Out 4.3 below.

Time-Out 4.3

The parent, adult and child in you

- What are the specific thoughts and reactions you have when you are under pressure? Assign a 'Parent', 'Adult' or 'Child' tag next to each of them.
- What are some counteractive Adult thoughts that will help you deal more effectively with the Parent and Child in you when under pressure?

Compare your reflections with the content of Figure 4.4. This resulted from an exercise with a managing director, Phoebe, who had become frustrated and disenchanted with circumstances in her work environment.

Figure 4.4 **Phoebe's thoughts, emotions and behaviours in the Parent, Adult and Child states.**

PARENT	
	'I'll do it for you'
	Pressure, worry – problems not shared
	Guilt – assuming blame for things not going right
	Disappointment – people don't live up to expectations
	Impose own ideas on people
	Judgemental
	'This is how it should be'
	Don't ask for help
ADULT	
	Sense of equality, sharing
	Open
	Confident, optimistic
	Belief – don't have to have answers
	Logical ('real' logic)
	Approachable
	Relaxed (sustainable)
	Considered
	Willing to accept help
CHILD	
	Hoping someone else sorts out my problems
	Victim, helpless
	Self-deprecating
	Don't take responsibility
	Short-sighted, rash decisions
	Not necessarily willing to be helped

By identifying and associating her thoughts, emotions and behaviours with the Parent, Adult and Child sides of herself, Phoebe recognised that she was operating outside her Adult state for the majority of the time, and that her decisions and actions were being determined mainly by her Parent or Child. This exercise helped Phoebe to identify times when she was not in her Adult state and to modify her thoughts and behaviour accordingly.

Over to Adrian . . .

In the late 1980s I was swimming in the US National Championships. This was a race that my coach and I had targeted as one in which I would attempt to break the World Record. About an hour before the race I remember walking outside for some fresh air as well as trying to calm down a bit. Next to the pool was a freeway with cars just whizzing past. I remember watching the cars. In one car I saw a woman with her children, and in another I saw a little old man, and I remember thinking about their lives in that moment. What were they doing? What was important to them? I imagined that they probably didn't even know that I was swimming that race, so why was I so worried about it? Millions of people couldn't care less! I started to realise it wasn't a big deal. To cope, I always think about the scale of what I'm trying to achieve and in the grand scheme of things, they aren't actually that important.

It's really quite fascinating when I look at Graham's comments about Transactional Analysis. I guess that being able to compete in a sport as a grown-up is really a continuation of the stuff you do at school. So, no surprise that you get all worked up when you don't win and your behaviour can seem a little childish.

My comments above would suggest that in the end, I was able to take an Adult view of racing. Interestingly, if I had taken my parents' view, then win or lose, I knew that I would still get a Chinese takeaway!

In business I deal with the pressures in the same way, it's actually more subconscious for me now. If something doesn't go the right way or I have a split second thought that we might not win an important piece of business, I just think differently about it. I learned most of these techniques by working with a coach (who was effectively my psychologist). They come as second nature to me, although I do occasionally seek guidance from a friend or colleague at work.

Asking For Help

Stress is often caused by thought patterns that are both negative and irrational. Furthermore, seeing a situation or another person's behaviour or attitude from another perspective can be difficult when you are so entrenched in your own perspective. Such circumstances often call for the input of a respected and trusted individual who can support you in developing other ways of viewing the world. Indeed, my research on mental toughness highlights 'seeking support when you need it' as a key attribute. This will require you to view asking for help as a strength rather than a weakness.

As emphasised above, the person(s) you choose to provide the support you may require to check out your thought patterns should first of all satisfy the 'respected' and 'trusted' criteria. They should also interact with you in their Adult state. The last thing you need is someone agreeing with the Child or Parent side of you. This will only exacerbate the stress you are experiencing. The best sources of support will be people who ask you questions as opposed to telling you how to think. Adult questions like 'on what evidence are your thoughts based?' will not only get you to think about the validity of your thoughts in a specific stress situation, but will also get you into the habit of asking yourself Adult questions in the future.

Tackling the situations and circumstances that cause you stress: situation-focused strategies

The most effective means of tackling stress, of course, is to address the source of the pressure that causes it. However, it is also often the most difficult of the coping strategies to implement. This factor, together with the frequent assumption and acceptance that little can be done about the pressure, means that many people never even consider this strategy until things get so serious that there is no alternative. Former rower and 1992 Olympic Gold Medal winner, Greg Searle, tells the story[17] of when he was having an occasional ache from a wisdom tooth. As a major competition approached, the pain became more consistent and severe and was a major distraction for him. He persevered with dealing with the symptoms for a couple of competitions before realising that more drastic action was required – he had the tooth taken out and banished that

[17] Personal communication, 2006.

particular stress forever. Unfortunately, not all strategies for coping with stress are as simple, straightforward and immediately effective, but it does illustrate the power and effectiveness of tackling the things that cause you stress head-on.

Situations that cause stress are typically associated with two factors that are too often common in any performance environment – lack of control and uncertainty. Nobody likes to feel out of control and unsure of what is expected of them. More specific factors that are particularly pertinent in both sport and business include role conflict, role uncertainty, interpersonal conflict, unrealistic performance targets, poor communication, demand overload, change, lack of time, poor management/leadership/coaching, and skills not being employed appropriately. This section deals with some strategies for dealing with situations like these.

Challenging assumptions

A key reason why situation-focused strategies are often ignored by people, who instead focus on dealing with their symptoms and appraisals, is that they often assume that they have no control or influence over the offending situation and so do not waste valuable time and effort in challenging 'the system'. The starting point is actually to challenge your assumptions before you are in a position to challenge the system. For example, do not assume that your manager will respond badly to feedback about how disempowered s/he makes you feel – s/he may respond very positively and be thankful that s/he has a means of forming a better relationship with you. And do not assume that unrealistic performance targets are not negotiable – indeed, the assumption of the goal-setter may be that they must be realistic because you have not challenged them!

Being assertive

Being assertive is not the same as being aggressive, awkward or ignoring others' needs. People who act assertively can often deal with situations in a relaxed and composed manner, avoiding misunderstandings and preventing themselves from being persuaded to act against their better judgement. Underlying the process of being assertive is your belief that all people are equal and have the same basic rights. In the case of role uncertainty, for example, explain to the people concerned how the uncertainty is making you feel and how it is impacting on your performance, and that you need your role to be clarified for the good of both yourself and the team.

Presenting some possible solutions rather than just the problem is often very helpful. At all times, respond in a non-aggressive, reasonable and self-assured fashion. This will give you the best chance of satisfying your need to address the source of the pressure in a constructive way.

Making decisions

It is often more difficult to make decisions when under stress. This can make things worse because dealing with stress often requires you to make decisions that will enable you to cope with it more effectively. For example, demand overload has the potential to leave you burned out if you don't tackle it. Decisions around how important success in your work is to you and what you are willing to commit, balanced against the other demands in your life, cannot be delayed if you are to deal with this source of stress effectively. Deciding how you will approach upcoming change rather than being a passive participant, and sometimes 'victim', can radically alter your experience of change.

If you are regularly missing out on selection for positions that you aspire to, then you have a decision to make about whether to move on or stick it out. Delaying such decisions merely prolongs the stress and the need to withstand its symptoms.

Maximising supports – minimising constraints

During my early career as a researcher at Sheffield University I was involved in a number of studies that examined stress levels and their causes in different occupations. One of these studies[18] involved spending time in a top security psychiatric hospital which housed patients who had committed some of the most horrendous crimes imaginable. Our task was to assess levels of stress in the mainly male nursing population and to uncover the major predictors. The predictors were placed into three different categories: the demands of the job, including their face-to-face dealings with some highly dangerous patients; the supports that helped them carry out the job; and the constraints that hindered them from doing their job.

The results revealed that the biggest predictor of stress in the nurses was constraints, followed by lack of supports and then demands. It was not the job itself that caused the stress; it was things like the slow decision-making

---

[18] K.Janman, G.Jones, R.Payne, & T.Rick. Some determinants of stress in psychiatric nurses. *International Journal of Nursing Studies*, 24, 129–144, 1987.

up the hierarchy and the things they were allowed and not allowed to do that were 'dictated by "suits" who had never been nurses'. We found a similar pattern of results in other occupations where stress was more related to the frustrations of the job and lack of support than doing the job itself.

The demands/supports/constraints approach provides a very useful framework for developing a structured situation-focused strategy for dealing with stress. With your own role in mind, use Time-Out 4.4 below to work through the process of identifying your demands, supports and constraints and reflect on the extent to which they impact on you.

Time-Out 4.4

DEMANDS, SUPPORTS, CONSTRAINTS

Demands

- Identify the demands on you in your role. This should include everything that is expected of you, and also things that underpin delivering against these expectations.

Supports

- Identify the supports that you have at your disposal to help satisfy these demands. Do not try to generate supports for each specific demand; instead, view the demands you have listed as a whole 'package'.
- Return to each support you have identified and rate on a 1 ('no support at all') to 10 ('total support') scale how much support you receive or derive from that particular support.

Constraints

- Identify the constraints that stop you satisfying the demands. Note that a support can also be a constraint. Again, do not try to generate constraints for each specific demand; instead, view the demands you have listed as a whole 'package'.
- Return to each constraint you have identified and rate how much influence you have over it on a 1 ('no influence') to 10 ('total influence') scale.

There is one other stage in this process – action planning. But before proceeding to this final stage, let's look at the output (shown in Figures 4.5 and 4.6) from two performers, one each from sport and business respectively, who have benefited from this exercise.

Case study

Peter, the sport performer in Figure 4.5, is a team sport player in his early 30s who is rated as one of the best players in the world in his particular position and role. The exercise proved to be an enlightening experience for Peter, because he realised there were several supports at his disposal that he was not really using. He also recognised that he had passively accepted constraints that he could have done something about. We used the output of the exercise as a means of developing a plan to deal with the sources of pressure and potential stress, as opposed to continuing to deal with symptoms. Several actions were identified which fitted into four key criteria:

1 they were in his control
2 they were realistic
3 they would make a 'real' impact, rather than merely 'paper over the cracks'
4 they would have an impact in a relatively short time frame.

Peter highlighted two constraints ('carrying too much weight' and 'waning desire to train') and one support ('nutritionist') as fitting these criteria, and the following actions were identified.

- Nutritionist - sit down with the nutritionist and develop a diet programme (this would also help with his weight concerns).
- Carrying too much weight - sit down with the fitness advisor and develop an updated personal training programme that would complement the training programme for the team as a whole.
- Waning desire to train - write down goals for weight loss and improvement on specific fitness tests regularly administered by the fitness advisor. Develop ways of introducing a 'fun' element into training.

Figure 4.5 Peter's demands, supports and constraints.

DEMANDS
- Train – give 100%
- Compete
- Earn money
- Travel
- Role model for young players
- Support younger players
- Deal with media
- Deal with sponsor
- Spend quality time with family
- Be successful

SUPPORTS (Rating)
- Wife and family (8)
- Mobile phone (9)
- Coach (8)
- Sponsor (7)
- Fitness advisor (6)
- Team-mates (6)
- Physiotherapist (9)
- Training facilities (8)
- Team manager (4)
- Match analyst (8)
- Nutritionist (2)
- Car (6)

CONSTRAINTS (Rating)
- Too many games (1)
- Depth of quality in squad (2)
- Governing body – don't understand the modern game (2)
- Sponsor – unreasonable demands on my time (3)
- Too much travelling – away from home too much (2)
- Young children – wake me up at night before games (3)
- Niggling injuries (5)
- Carrying too much weight (8)
- Waning desire to train (10)
- Constantly in public eye (3)

Case study

Freya, the business performer in Figure 4.6, is in her late 30s and is a board director of a large global business organisation. We worked through the same procedure described above, focusing on tackling sources of pressure that caused her stress, and arrived at one support ('direct reports') and two constraints ('MD - slow decision-making' and 'lack of time') that Freya would develop actions around. The actions were as follows.

- Direct reports - organise one-to-one meetings with direct reports to explore how the relationships can be more mutually supportive.
- MD - slow decision-making - meet with the MD to explain how his timely decision-making is key to her performing her role effectively. Enquire how she can support the MD in making decisions, e.g. providing him with more information, etc.
- Lack of time - talk to her Personal Assistant about organising blocks of time for meetings and blocks of her 'own time' when she is unavailable for meetings.

Figure 4.6 Freya's demands, supports and constraints.

DEMANDS
- Delivering the numbers
- Communicate strategy
- Challenge people to deliver
- Report to the MD
- Work with fellow directors
- Inspire people
- Keep shareholders happy
- Establish good work-life balance

SUPPORTS (Rating)
- Direct reports (6)
- Personal Assistant (7)
- Email (7)
- Laptop computer (9)
- Partner (8)
- MD (5)
- Performance management reviews (6)
- Budget (6)

CONSTRAINTS (Rating)
- Email – too many (3)
- Quiet market (1)
- Shareholder expectations – too unrealistic (1)
- Lack of time (2)
- Some direct reports – poor people managers (4)
- New IT system – 'bugs' (2)
- MD – slow decision-making (3)
- Open plan working – too much noise (3)
- Too much travel – tiring (4)

Identifying demands, supports and constraints is a simple and effective way of developing a situation-focused strategy for dealing with stress. It helps performers who have previously lost sight of how much control and influence they really have over factors that they have assumed they could do little about. Freya had 'learned' to accept that she could do nothing about her lack of time or her MD's slow decision-making. This exercise enabled her to recognise that she did have some control and her actions resulted in a significant reduction in her stress.

Now return to your own demands, supports and constraints you identified and recorded in Time-Out 4.4. Work through Time-Out 4.5 below to arrive at an action plan for maximising your supports and minimising the constraints on you.

Time-Out 4.5

Demands, supports and constraints action plan

Go back to Time-Out 4.4 and have a look at the supports that you did *not* rate as a '10' in terms of the level of support you currently receive. Using the criteria below, choose one or two that you would like to work on.

- It should be in your *control* to do something about it.
- The changes you wish to make should be *realistic*.
- Any changes you make will have a *'real' impact*, rather than merely 'paper over the cracks'
- Any changes will have an impact in a relatively *short time frame*.

List the supports to work on and record any actions you intend to take.

Now go to the constraints in Time-Out 4.4 and have a look at the ones you did not score a '1' on in terms of the level of control or influence you have. Using the same criteria, select one or two that you would like to work on. List the constraints and record any actions you intend to take.

Like any action plan, it will only be as good as what you do with it. It's now up to you to make things happen in order to maximise your supports and minimise your constraints. It could make a big difference!

Over to Adrian . . .

Looking at the stress-coping model and its application to my working life, I realise that one of my biggest areas of focus has been to challenge the sources of pressure. In business, market forces are usually out of your control, but obviously some companies survive and some don't. I'm pretty sure that a key factor has to be the approach towards it. Those that survive, and indeed thrive, do so because of a leadership group who take initiative, and control what they are able to, instead of bemoaning the current situation and always taking defensive positions.

Some of this basic learning started out in swimming; for example if there are a lot of waves in the pool, realising there's nothing I can do about it! All I can control is my stroke and adapting it to cope with the waves (and in terms of appraisal, recognising that it's the same for everyone and someone has to win the race).

I have seen mentally tough people, particularly in business, who seem able to recognise their constraints, and not only minimise the impact of them, but even appreciate that they can do something about them.

Maximising your supports is equally important. I have always known that you don't achieve much by doing it all by yourself! It took me a bad Olympics to realise that it wasn't being tough to stand alone and forge ahead. Rather, that to achieve something so huge, I had to draw on all the expertise available to me. From being a team of two in 1984 (myself and my swim coach), in 1988 it became a support group of swimming coach, strength coach, nutritionist, psychologist, physiotherapist and sponsors!

It didn't even take me one day of being in business to realise that you don't do it by yourself. I wouldn't have even contemplated starting up a business without the support of my fellow founders!

Chris Andy Scott Emma Studies

Chris

Chris' inquisitive intellect meant that he was keen to understand what was happening to him. He worked through the stress and coping model, and realised that the situation had got the better of him and that this was where he needed to begin the process of becoming his own man again; to make decisions he believed in rather than decisions he thought were expected and demanded of him. The demands/supports/constraints framework proved particularly beneficial to Chris, emphasising who and what his supports were and how he had lost sight of them. He identified who were important supports in helping him make key decisions. It also allowed him to see that he had been passively accepting constraints that he actually had a degree of control over. The situation had become much clearer to him and he began the process of assuming control again.

Chris also realised that he needed some time to himself. He was showing early signs of burnout and he resolved to schedule time-outs into his working week and to spend more time with his family. This was a symptom-focused strategy aimed at allowing his mind to switch off from the pressure he was under.

Andy

Andy quickly recognised that his stress was self-imposed and that his appraisal of circumstances and how others perceived him was distorted to the extent that he viewed almost every situation as threatening. Acknowledging the choice he had over how to perceive his world and the people in it, Andy worked hard at seeing opportunities to build respect and good working relationships with his colleagues. He began to see how he could actually derive some pleasure and enjoyment from his new role.

As part of this process, it also dawned on Andy that he had perfectionist tendencies that accounted for him never being able to live up to his own expectations. This was an important realisation that helped him to understand the situation he found himself in and how to deal with it.

Scott

Scott was not interested in models - he wanted a quick fix! He worked primarily on a strategy aimed at helping him deal with his stress symptoms. He learned all three forms (deep, intermediate and quick) of meditative relaxation to help him with his intense symptoms of stress before and during tournaments. Scott found the quick version particularly helpful in helping him to clear his mind and stay in the 'here and now' during competitive rounds. He also worked on trying to reduce the pressure he imposed on himself by his mounting expectations (i.e. appraisal) as his situation worsened.

Scott had created a mindset that was based on an 'I must win this next tournament' mentality, but this was not actually the case. In fact, a few good performances in which he made it to the last two days (i.e. the 'cut') of tournaments would be sufficient. He worked on allowing his Adult to put ▶

things in perspective and to see how they really were. This enabled Scott to realise that he had more control over circumstances than he had previously imagined and that he needed to think in terms of putting in some good performances rather than on winning.

Emma

Emma's stress was caused not by being a woman in a male-dominated environment, but how she thought females in senior positions were viewed. Her realisation that she was attempting to be something and someone other than the person who had been appointed to the role was core to dealing with the situation. Emma's perception and appraisal of the situation was influencing her thoughts and her interactions with colleagues. She began the process of challenging her own assumptions about how a female in a senior position was generally perceived by male colleagues.

Emma identified a male colleague she respected and trusted who she would approach to 'check out' the validity of her assumptions. He actually turned into being a valuable source of day-to-day support over the next few months. She also looked at how the situation was influencing her behaviours and how these were impacting on both herself and others. Emma was addressing both her symptoms and appraisal in a manner that would make a difference in the short and longer term.

In a nutshell

- There are two sides to pressure; it can exhilarate and energise, and it can drain and crush performers.
- The negative response to pressure is stress.
- Stress is not always caused by major events; it can simply be the result of the daily grind, hassles and sometimes monotony of work.
- The key to controlling your stress to manageable proportions is to be aware of when you are stressed.
- The way you are as a person and your past history (i.e. your predisposition) is a big factor in determining how you respond to pressure and the likelihood of becoming stressed.
- Negative appraisals of situations and circumstances are likely to result in stress, but remember that you have a choice over how you appraise things so that most stress is self-imposed.
- Symptoms of stress can be broken down into mental, physical and behavioural categories. Be aware of subtle changes in your thoughts, bodily response and behaviour in helping you to recognise that you are stressed.
- There are three basic options open to you in dealing with stress: addressing and controlling the symptoms; reappraising the negative thoughts that result in stress; tackling the things that cause you stress.

What next?

- Experiment with some relaxation techniques and make appropriate behavioural changes to help you deal with your symptoms of stress.
- Take an Adult perspective and seek support from respected and trusted others to challenge the way you appraise situations and circumstances that cause you stress.
- Tackle the things that cause you stress head-on. Challenge your assumptions about what is possible. Maximise your supports and minimise your constraints.

5 Staying Strong in Your Self-Belief

After reading this chapter you will know about:

- The key difference between self-esteem and self-confidence
- How to accept, respect and trust yourself
- How to be confident about being successful in specific situations and circumstances

Self-belief is an essential part of the make-up of the very best performers I have come across. And elite sport performers involved in our research ranked self-belief in their abilities and in being able to achieve their goals as the number one attribute of mental toughness. Ongoing research carried out at Lane4 is revealing a similar pattern in mentally tough executives. But what is self-belief, and how do you develop it so that it remains robust and impenetrable under pressure? This chapter explores and delves deeply into this crucial pillar of mental toughness and will provide an enlightening way forward for enhancing your own self-belief.

Over to Adrian . . .

In the end it simply boils down to these facts: when I thought I was going to win, I usually did; when I thought I was going to lose, I always did. Throughout the years my belief wavered. As a boy of 14 it was shaky at best. Successive victories and a rapid ascent to the ranks as one of the world's best swimmers built a stronger platform. Going into the business world I had no real proof that I could make it, but a strong belief in my personal qualities as a performer.

What does self-belief look and sound like?

Self-belief at its strongest and most robust is accompanied by a humility that sets mentally tough people aside from others whose self-belief is perhaps a little more fragile. They do not take things personally and see negative feedback only as a means of moving further forward in their development. They have no need to inform others of their own achievements because they possess an inner belief that requires no external reinforcement to sustain it. Of course, these performers have doubts from time to time, but this is mainly about their confidence in specific situations and can actually serve an important purpose – it prevents them from becoming complacent.

The deep inner belief that these performers possess allows them to operate in a way that engenders consistent high performance. It does this in a number of ways, including their desire and ability to:

- set and achieve stretching goals;
- take and learn from criticism;
- establish a balanced perspective on strengths and weaknesses, and to tackle the weaknesses head on;
- take risks;
- make decisions without fear of being wrong;
- control potentially debilitating fear;
- bounce back from setbacks with renewed focus and effort;
- create a positive future;
- perhaps most importantly in the context of mental toughness, provide them with a strong foundation for dealing with pressure.

Then there are those performers who 'appear' to have strong self-belief. They are often keen to tell you how strong their self-belief is and how much ability they have. They have a need to verbalise and externalise it because they are probably trying to convince themselves as well as seeking external reinforcement from people who will hopefully agree with them. These performers' self-belief is more exposed and vulnerable than those performers referred to earlier.

There are others who are very aware of their lack of self-belief. I have encountered a number of performers in both sport and business who are very good at what they do, but have struggled to scale the dizzy heights of achievement because of their lack of true self-belief. These include senior executives, amongst them MDs, more than one of whom have informed me behind closed doors that they are 'waiting to be found out' and have been 'lucky' to get where they are. They tend to be highly self-conscious, self-critical and often have distorted and negative perceptions about what others think of them and their ability. They begin each working day with a self-imposed handicap that exacerbates any pressure they are under. I have also worked with sport performers whose lack of self-belief is an obstacle to taking risks, testing their limits or withstanding the dark side of pressure. Some of these have been so handicapped that they have fallen way below achieving their potential.

Over to Adrian . . .

In swimming the one occasion when your belief (or lack of it!) is most tested is in that 'ready room' half an hour before you go out to race. You sit with your fellow finalists preparing for the upcoming battle. Most of the time I kept to myself, but occasionally would look around to see how my rivals were faring. Some were quite passive, focusing inwards and betraying no signs of lack of belief. They seemed to have a calm exterior. Others would be quite the opposite, with energy pouring out of everywhere, nervously jiggling their arms or legs. At those times when our eyes met, I could see the fear, and indeed the dismantling of their own belief. I imagined them looking at me and reflecting on my successes in a resigned way, rather than building their own as a suit of armour. They were already beaten.

Self-belief is, therefore, one of the key factors underpinning high performance. Fortunately, it is not an attribute that you either have or you haven't – it can be worked on and developed to levels that deliver extraordinary performance.

What is self-belief?

Self-belief comprises two key components – self-esteem and self-confidence. Their relationship is best understood via the use of a metaphor. Think of self-belief as a rose, with roots that grow unseen below the earth, and leaves and petals that are the part of the rose exposed to environmental conditions above the ground. When the roots are well-nourished the leaves and petals are healthy and flourish. Conversely, when the roots are deprived of water for a protracted period, the leaves and petals will whither and wilt. The shorter term health of the leaves and petals will also depend on the ever-changing environment above the ground. In conditions that are not to the rose's liking, such as extreme heat, the leaves and petals will suffer; in more congenial conditions, the rose's leaves and petals will thrive.

The roots represent your **self-esteem**, or how you value yourself as a human being. Self-esteem is a way of thinking and feeling that implies that you accept, respect and trust yourself. It is developed over time and is unlikely to alter very much in the short term. It is largely unaffected by the external environment so that it is within your control. The leaves and petals of the rose represent your **self-confidence**. Self-confidence reflects your optimism about being successful in specific situations and circumstances. This is the part of your belief that is at the mercy of the changing environment; it is more easily and immediately influenced by external conditions so that you are not always in control of it and it can fluctuate significantly over a very short time period. Essentially, you hand over your self-confidence to others, or situational conditions, to determine its level and nature.

Imagine you are making a presentation, and as you look around individual faces in the audience your confidence rises as you see someone who is smiling and nodding in agreement at the points you are making. Now imagine what happens to your confidence as your gaze turns to a person whose expression cannot hide her obvious boredom and disinterest, and then to another individual who clearly does not like what you are saying. Notice any difference in your confidence?

The key to your confidence, therefore, is that it is dictated by things in the external environment that are largely outside your control. However, there is also another important predictor of confidence that is totally within your control – self-esteem. The health of the leaves and petals of a rose are affected by external conditions, but they ultimately depend on the health of the roots for their survival. When the roots are healthy so are the leaves and petals, and vice versa. The relationship in the context of self-esteem and self-confidence is shown in Figure 5.1. When self-esteem is relatively low, self-confidence fluctuates at a relatively low level; when self-esteem is relatively high, self-confidence fluctuates at a relatively high level.

Figure 5.1 The relationship between self-esteem and self-confidence.

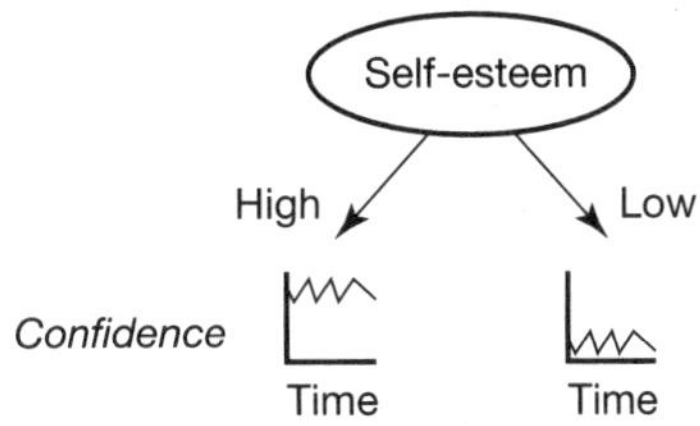

My experience of working with people who wish to enhance their self-belief is that their natural tendency is to focus on improving their self-confidence. My general approach is to get performers working firstly on their self-esteem before tackling techniques to build their confidence. In this way, as important performances get closer they focus more on their ability and what they have achieved over the long term than on factors in the environment that they cannot control.

Over to Adrian . . .

When things are tough for me I always draw on my inner strength, mainly calling on past experiences of having been in difficult situations and having come through. I have so many reasons to feel good about the resources I have. I (perhaps obviously) have a strength based on my swimming achievements. This part of my life will always be with me, even though it doesn't really help me in business to be able to swim fast! It does make me feel good to remember past successes. I also assume that the environment I am in, no matter what the field of endeavour, will be at times harsh – but that it can also be good. I keep on looking inside to manage myself through.

Developing self-esteem

The fundamental factor to bear in mind when implementing strategies for developing self-esteem is that it comes from within. The basis for your feelings of self-worth is internal so that how you feel about yourself is within your control. There is no quick pathway to building self-esteem that is durable and stable. The robust self-esteem that is required to make you mentally tough will not develop overnight or as a consequence of a single action, thought, decision or behavioural change. Instead, self-esteem is enhanced gradually and through a number of different strategies described in the following pages.

Giving yourself some credit

Think back to a recent success or a time when things went well for you. Why did you succeed? Was it because you are good at what you do, or perhaps because you put a lot of effort into it? Was it because it was easy for you to succeed, or perhaps because you were lucky?

Now think back to a recent failure or a time when things went against you. Why did it happen? Was it because you were not good enough, or perhaps because you did not try hard enough? Was it because it was too difficult for you, or perhaps because you were unlucky? Record your reflections on Time-Out 5.1.

Time-Out 5.1

Developing self-esteem 1

Giving yourself some credit

- Think back to a recent success or a time when things went well for you. Why did you succeed?
- Think back to a recent failure or when things went against you. Why did it happen?

There may be other causes of your success or failure but, whatever you attribute them to, the attributions will fall within two dimensions:

- an internal-external dimension that reflects whether the cause or 'source of control' is internal or external to you;
- and a constant-variable dimension that reflects the degree of 'change-ability' of the cause.

Figure 5.2[19] shows how 'ability' is an internal factor that is under your control, but it is also a constant factor that cannot be changed to any great extent in the short term. 'Effort' is internal since it is under your total control, and it is also variable so that you can change how much effort you put in very quickly. 'Performance difficulty' is external in that it is largely determined by others or the environment you are performing in and it is also constant so that you can do little to change it. 'Luck' is clearly external and variable since you have no control over it and it can change very rapidly.

Figure 5.2 How do you attribute success and failure?

CHANGEABILITY \ SOURCE OF CONTROL	INTERNAL	EXTERNAL
CONSTANT	(1) Ability Expertise Experience Skills	(3) Performance difficulty Tools to perform Team members' capability Quality of opposition/competition Targets set by others Incentives
VARIABLE	(2) Effort Practice Preparation Planning Own thoughts, attitudes, emotions	(4) Luck Performance conditions (weather, marketplace, etc) Others' thoughts, attitudes, emotions

Figure 5.2 also shows other causes of success and failure that fall within each of the quadrants emanating from the combination of the internal-external and constant-variable dimensions. The major point of interest in the context of enhancing self-esteem is the **internal-constant quadrant**

[19] This figure is based on the work of B. Weiner, *Theories of Motivation: From Mechanism to Cognition*, Rand-McNally, 1972.

(1). This includes causes such as your ability, expertise, experience and skills that are totally under your control, and are constant and enduring. If you have a success and attribute the cause to one or more of these things then this will instil an enduring sense of pride, competence and optimism in you that will feed your self-esteem. You can essentially feel good about yourself in a way that will not disappear overnight.

The downside of course, is that when you attribute failure to things that are internal and constant, you are likely to feel bad about yourself for reasons that are difficult to change in the short-term. This is bound to threaten your sense of self-worth, although it is important to remember that the durable and stable nature of self-esteem means that it will take a number of successes/failures to be attributed in this way before self-esteem is significantly affected either way. In other words, your self-esteem should not be affected by one very good or very bad performance, but rather by successive incidents that serve to continually reinforce your thoughts and feelings about your self-worth.

At the other extreme is the **external-variable quadrant** (4) which includes causes of success and failure that you have no control over and are variable (e.g. luck, performance conditions and others' thoughts, attitudes and emotions). These attributions should have no impact on your self-esteem since they have nothing to do with you as a person.

Similarly, the causes of success or failure in the **external-constant quadrant** (3) are about other people and the environment you are performing in so that they should have relatively little impact on your self-esteem (e.g. performance difficulty, tools to perform, team members' capability, quality of opposition/competition, targets set by others, incentives).

The **internal-variable quadrant** (2) does include causes that are under your control (e.g. effort, practice, preparation, planning, own thoughts, attitudes, emotions), but their variable nature means they are likely to have less impact on self-esteem than attributions made in the internal-constant quadrant (1).

The key message, therefore, is that self-esteem can be developed and enhanced by finding aspects of success that are attributable to the more permanent and enduring aspects of yourself, such as your ability and experience. Performers I have worked with who have had relatively low self-esteem have often struggled to take personal credit for their successes. The successes have been because they 'were in the right place at the right time', or perhaps they were 'part of an outstanding team'.

ikewise, they have 'wanted' to attribute failures to their own shortcomings and mistakes. For example, I have been working hard with one particular MD with relatively low self-esteem on strategies that will prevent him from apologising for everything that goes wrong in his organisation and giving anyone else bar himself the plaudits for the successes. Another real challenge has been working closely with a young team sport player who felt he had no right to be on the same field as older players he had idolised from an early age. Much of the work with these particular performers has been on working out how they have got to the level they are performing at and attributing it to internal factors such as ability, skills, etc.

Over to Adrian . . .

To reflect back on the point Graham made above on taking credit for your own successes, I can't help but think that this is one of the most critical aspects of building self-belief. At my most fragile I found it difficult to hold on to these past successes, and worse than that, I thought it would be somehow arrogant to think that I was 'great' because of something I had done.

During my childhood we were brought up to believe that arrogance and superiority were highly unattractive qualities. I still think this is right, but it can be a filter to how we think of our success. Getting beyond that to a place where I would walk out to a race believing I would win, that I was better than my rivals, was difficult but ultimately became my biggest strength. I am sure that I started to attribute these successes to my own abilities (i.e. the internal-constant quadrant) and I got over my own internal resistance. I no longer see it as arrogance, but a very important piece in holding on to my self-worth.

Now return to the attributions you made for your own success and failure in Time-Out 5.1 and work through the exercise in Time-Out 5.2 below to help you better understand how they fit into the Source of Control/Changeability framework described above.

Time-Out 5.2

How do you attribute sucess and failure?

Think back to the reasons you gave for your success and failure in Time-Out 5.1 and place each of them in the appropriate quadrant in the attribution framework: see sample below.

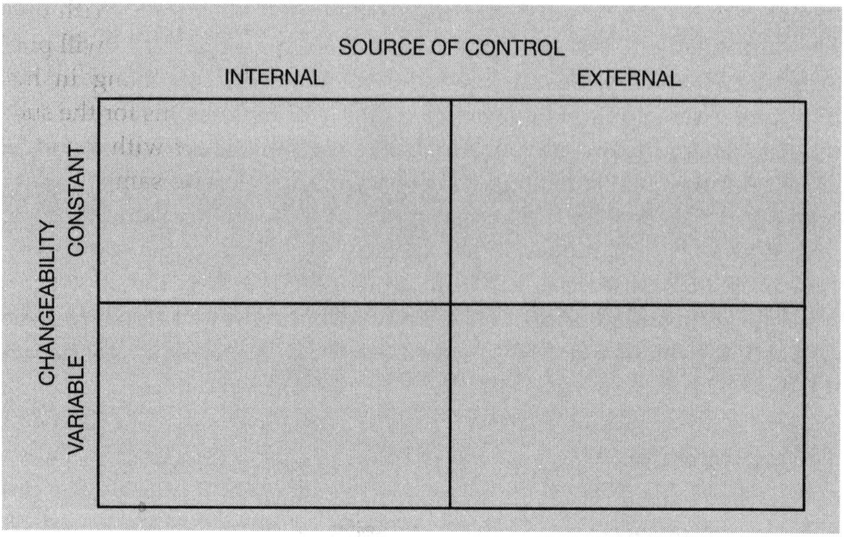

Do you typically attribute causes in this way? This will give you a strong indication as to how your attributions impact on your sense of self-worth. The key to the whole process is to take appropriate personal credit for your successes and not to distort your attributions of failure in a way that you assume personal responsibility when it is unjustified. Underlying this message is the need to be logical and rational in the way you attribute success and failure. Kidding yourself will serve no long-term benefit and may even prevent you from developing as a performer because you ignore key development areas.

Establishing and reinforcing your worth

Do you spend time thinking about your self-worth? Not very often? It probably takes too long, it's too hard and you are not sure why you are doing it in the first place. The likely fallback position is that you often rely on your most recent past experiences to gauge 'how you are doing' in life. But robust self-esteem is not based on the last few days, weeks or even months – it is based on your whole experience as a human being, from early childhood to now. Use Time-Out 5.3 below to think about your life to date.

Time-Out 5.3

Developing self-esteem 2

Life achievements

Reflect on and list your achievements in life.

Now examine the list you have generated and get a feel for the nature of the content. Are the achievements mainly, or exclusively, tangible things? (By 'tangible' I mean things you can touch, see, point to, provide a certificate as evidence, etc; in other words things that are measurable). My experience of performers carrying out this exercise is that they find it relatively easy to list tangible achievements, but often dry up when thinking about non-tangible ones. Figure 5.3 shows the initial output from two performers: Liz, a 37 year-old who had achieved senior executive status at a relatively young age in the context of the organisation where she is employed; and Evie, a 26 year-old team sport player who has been playing at international level for seven years.

Both approached me about strategies for improving their confidence levels. Liz's confidence was dented when she perceived her ability to be under question; for example, when colleagues challenged some of the decisions she made. Evie's confidence dropped after disappointing personal performances and reading critical reports in the media. In both cases we discussed the importance of building robust self-esteem to 'protect' against threats to their confidence, and embarked on establishing and reinforcing their worth as human beings rather than 'just' very good

Figure 5.3 Liz's and Evie's initial list of achievements.

Liz	Evie
• *MBA*	• *Capped 48 times for country*
• *Promoted three times in last five years*	• *First cap at 19*
• *Youngest person to achieve a senior leadership role*	• *Appointed team captain two years ago*
• *Grown a business to a profit of £1.1 million*	• *Player of the Year twice*
• *Passed driving test first time*	• *Two A levels*

performers. Figure 5.3 shows that the output from their first attempts at listing their achievements comprised tangible outcomes. Despite the impressive nature of both lists, the highly visible nature of them meant that they were essentially measuring their worth against society's expectations and values – they were successful in comparison to other people.

True and robust self-esteem is about recognising your inherent worth in such a way that you do not compare yourself with other people. The next stage of the process, therefore, involved moving them beyond tangible achievements to identifying achievements that were non-tangible. Do this for yourself in Time-Out 5.4 below.

Time-Out 5.4

Achievements continued

Add any non-tangible achievements that you have not included in the list in Time-Out 5.3.

You might have found that quite difficult. Both Liz and Evie found it strange to think about achievements that are not measurable and needed some encouragement to 'think deep'. Eventually, they surprised themselves by generating things, shown in Figure 5.4, that they considered achievements but had not previously thought of as such. Liz recognised that her peers constantly sought her advice on difficult issues, that she

Figure 5.4 Liz's and Evie's deeper reflections on their achievements.

Liz:	**Evie:**
Tangible achievements	**Tangible achievements**
• *MBA*	• *Capped 48 times for country*
• *Promoted three times in last five years*	• *First cap at 19*
• *Youngest person to achieve a senior leadership role*	• *Appointed team captain two years ago*
• *Grown a business to a profit of £1.1million*	• *Player of the Year twice*
• *Passed driving test first time*	• *Two A levels*

Non-tangible achievements	Non-tangible achievements
• *Source of advice for peers*	• *Gritty way I came back after a serious injury*
• *Good team player*	• *Good leader, supportive*
• *Have established an open and honest culture in my part of the business*	• *Popular with supporters*
• *Happily married*	• *Coped well with parents' divorce*

was a good team player, had created an open and honest working environment and was happily married. Evie recalled the gritty way she had come back after quite a serious injury as a significant achievement, in addition to being a good leader and someone who was popular with the team's supporters. She also recognised that she had coped well with her parents' divorce during her teens.

The next stage was to dig even deeper, and to focus on the tangible achievements and what they provided 'evidence of', and then on the non-tangible achievements and what they were 'underpinned by'. The output of this stage is shown in Figure 5.5(a) and (b). Both performers recognised how their tangible achievements were a reflection of their personal competence, and that the non-tangible achievements were underpinned by core attributes and values (e.g. care for others, integrity, wisdom) that are an enduring part of them. Together, these formed the building blocks for their self-esteem.

Figure 5.5 (a) What Liz's tangible achievements provide evidence of and what her non-tangible achievements are underpinned by.

Liz:

Tangible Achievements	Evidence of
• *MBA*	• *Knowledge*
• *Promoted three times in last five years*	• *Personal competence*
• *Youngest person to achieve a senior leadership role*	• *Talent*
• *Grown a business to a profit of £1.1 million*	• *Business competence*
• *Passed driving test first time*	• *Quick learner*

Non-tangible achievements	Underpinned by
• *Source of advice for peers*	• *Wisdom*
• *Good team player*	• *Collaboration*
• *Have established an open and honest culture in my part of the business*	• *Integrity*
• *Happily married*	• *Capacity to share and compromise*

Figure 5.5 (b) What Evie's tangible achievements provide evidence of and what her non-tangible achievements are underpinned by.

Evie:

Tangible achievements	Evidence of
• *Capped 48 times for country*	• *Experience*
• *First cap at 19*	• *Talent*
• *Appointed team captain two years ago*	• *Leadership*
• *Player of the Year twice*	• *Ability*
• *Two A levels*	• *Academic intellect*
Non-tangible achievements	**Underpinned by**
• *Gritty way I came back after a serious injury*	• *Determination*
• *Good leader, supportive*	• *Care for others*
• *Popular with supporters*	• *Likeable*
• *Coped well with parents' divorce*	• *Resilience*

Now go to the tangible achievements *you* have identified and think about what they provide evidence of. And think about what underpins each of your non-tangible achievements. Set aside a decent amount of time to do this and record your conclusions in Time-Out 5.5 below.

Time-Out 5.5

What lies beneath your achievements

- List the tangible achievements you identified in Time-Out 5.3 and then think about what they provide evidence of.
- Now list your non-tangible achievements identified in Time-Outs 5.3 and 5.4 and think about what they are underpinned by. If you find yourself struggling with this, then think about what it is about you that has enabled this achievement.

The attributes and values you have generated form the building blocks of your own self-esteem. You may need to remind yourself of them from time to time. Many of the performers I have worked with have written them on small cards they carry around in their organisers or kit bags. They are there for them when they find themselves in pressured situations that threaten their confidence, when factors in the external environment are impacting negatively on their thoughts and feelings. The words on the cards allow them to step back inside themselves in order to regain control and gather strength from their self-esteem.

In this way feelings of anxiety and doubt about presenting to a particularly challenging audience, for example, can be over-ridden by thoughts about your competence and knowledge demonstrated over a long period, together with enduring attributes and values that will serve you well in this particular situation. Remember, your worth is a function of you as a person and not the circumstances that surround you!

Letting go of perfectionist tendencies

This section is really for those of you who have perfectionist tendencies, but will be useful anyway because my experience of high achievers is that they all have some elements of perfectionism in them. Perfectionism can be thought of in terms of a tendency to routinely set expectations for yourself and others that are unrealistically high. Perfectionists also tend to focus on small flaws and shortcomings in themselves and their achievements and ignore what is good about them. Perfectionism has already appeared in this book as being important in contributing to stress. It is also a common cause of reduced self-esteem because perfectionism directs a performer's focus to those small flaws and shortcomings in themselves. Their often unrealistic expectations mean that nothing they do is ever good enough and they are highly critical of themselves.

Overcoming perfectionism requires a fundamental shift in your attitude towards yourself and how you approach life in general. The following strategies and guidelines provide a starting point for this shift.

Celebrating your achievements

I knew one performer who had achieved some impressive things in his career, but told me that he was 'disgusted at his lack of achievement' when he compared them with a very small number of extremely high achievers. The important message from this anecdote is that it is important that you learn to celebrate your achievements, and focus in particular on those that are non-tangible, since these are the achievements that are not gauged against society's expectations, and are underpinned by attributes and values that are at the core of you. These are the source of being able to feel good about yourself as a human being, if only you allow yourself to recognise, accept and place value in them.

Accepting fallibility

Nobody is perfect so why should *you* expect to be? You will never achieve this goal. The problem with performers with perfectionist tendencies is that they appear almost compelled to focus on the smallest flaws and mistakes and to 'beat themselves up' over them. The best performers accept that they will mess up from time to time. Indeed, learning from making mistakes is an important part of their development. The crucial element is to dwell on mistakes for only as long as it takes to draw out the important learning points, and then to move on and to focus on the here-and-now.

Focusing on process as well as outcome

It would be unrealistic of me to suggest that you should not focus on outcomes such as winning and promotions. However, there can only ever be one winner and not everyone can be promoted. This means that focusing on the processes that underpin outcomes is important, and for two reasons. Firstly, you may not win or get promoted, but you can still perform well at the processes and derive some satisfaction from that. Secondly, focusing solely on outcomes only adds to the pressure that you are under as a result of your strong need to achieve. Focusing on processes can alleviate the pressure to some extent.

Setting realistic goals

This is a lot easier said than done when you have perfectionist tendencies. Perfectionists' goals are rarely met since they are so high, but they struggle to accept that their goals should be set any lower. You will need to identify any constraints on you, such as time and lack of control over some important factors in the environment, and also personal limitations. This may need the help of someone you respect and trust, in order to be able to set expectations that are attainable.

Recognising and overcoming perfectionist thinking styles

There are essentially three types of perfectionist thinking styles[20]:

1 Should/must thinking:	'I should be able to do this right'
	'I must not mess up'
2 All-or-nothing thinking:	'I can't do this at all'
	'This is completely wrong'
3 Overgeneralisation thinking:	'I'll never be able to do this'
	'I'll always get things wrong'

Recognising when you are engaging in such thoughts and self-talk is the starting point. This is particularly important when you are under pressure because such self-talk only serves to exacerbate the pressure. Recognise your use of 'should', 'must', 'never', 'have to' and 'always' when you are under pressure and learn to develop counter-statements that are more rational and positive. The process of changing self-talk is described later in this chapter.

[20] Edmund J. Bourne, *The Anxiety and Phobia Workbook*, New Harbinger Publications, Oakland, California, 1995.

Over to Adrian . . .

I was quite a shy and introverted child. I was happy in my own space, but seemed to find it hard to become part of the 'in-crowd' at school. My academic achievements were also, in the main, average. It appeared that I was just about average at most sports. I had learned to swim, as every child does, to save my own life should I fall in to the water. But it wasn't until the age of 8 that I had my first swimming race.

Not only did this feed the need for personal endeavour, but I also seemed to be above average. I started to feel good about myself. Winning the Airedale and Wharfedale one-length backstroke for under 9s was the best thing that had happened to me in my short life. Looking back on it now, I know that building on this achievement with other swimming-related success was the key to me building a strong self-worth. In fact, I am sure that the main reason that I dedicated myself wholeheartedly to swimming was because it was practically the only way I was building self-esteem. It gave me something to feel good about.

I remember telling my coach when I was 14 about my dreams to win the Olympics, and quite cleverly he had me hold on to this dream, but break it down to more achievable targets. At such a young age, I had been coached to set short and medium-term targets. In parallel with this, I learned the other golden rule about goal setting, and that was that all achievements are made at the process level. Our entire daily swimming training sessions focused solely on the various kicking and pulling techniques, drills and stroke work, as well as dives and turns. I spent four months trying to spin round the wall faster!

Where do you start?

You have probably 'lived' with your current level of self-esteem for quite a while. So if you want to improve it, you will need to be patient and work on it gradually. The strategies and techniques described in this section provide a framework within which you can start to enhance your self-esteem. The framework essentially involves three processes that you may wish to follow:

1 Recognising how you typically attribute success and failure and how this impacts upon your self-esteem.

2 Getting to the abilities, beliefs and values that lie at the core of you via careful consideration of both your tangible and non-tangible achievements.

3 Recognising and letting go of any perfectionist tendencies.

Developing self-confidence

There will be times when you neither have time, nor is it appropriate, to reflect on your worth as a human being and you need to be able to tweak or significantly raise your confidence to meet the demands of specific situations. As I stated earlier in this chapter, even the very best performers have self-doubts from time to time when in highly pressured situations. They have therefore developed strategies for quickly regaining and enhancing confidence levels. These strategies are best understood within the context of a framework of situation-specific self-confidence[21] in which confidence is a function of four factors:

- focusing on recent performance accomplishments;
- drawing on own and others' experiences;
- managing self-talk;
- interpreting your readiness to perform in a positive way.

Research has consistently shown these factors to be important predictors of success in skilled performers. In addition, research findings show that they aid performers' commitment to highly challenging goals, as well as increasing persistence and effort that enables them to bounce back after setbacks. Importantly in the context of dealing with pressure, self-confidence also appears to protect performers against the negative effects of anxiety.[22] The strategies and techniques described below are therefore based on the framework of self-confidence described above.

---

[21] Albert Bandura, Self-Efficacy: Toward a Unifying Theory of Behavioural Change, *Psychological Review*, 84, 191–215, 1977.

[22] Graham Jones & Lew Hardy (Eds), *Stress and Performance in Sport*, Wiley, 1995, p. 273.

Focusing on recent performance accomplishments

Unlike self-esteem, which is based on achievements over a long time frame, self-confidence in specific situations is governed by much more recent accomplishments, say over the past few weeks or perhaps months. What have been your own accomplishments over the last few weeks and months? Are you able to recall them easily? Reminding yourself of them when your confidence is becoming a little fragile is an effective strategy for bolstering it when under pressure.

This has significant implications for setting goals. You probably have long-term goals related to your performance ambitions, but have you broken them down into medium- and short-term goals? The short-term goals are particularly important in the context of enhancing confidence, since if you achieve them you can regularly gain confidence from seeing them accomplished. This will allow you to build up a store of recent performance accomplishments which you may wish to record on a small card and carry around with you for use when you need a confidence boost.

You will also have a record of your recent accomplishments in the form of a mental image. Try replaying one or two of them to see how vivid they are. Imagine all details of the accomplishment, including the performance itself and how it made you feel. Imagery is a very powerful technique and can be of enormous benefit. Store these images up and replay them to bolster your confidence before important events. Use Time-Out 5.6 below to begin to build up your 'store' of performance accomplishments.

Time-Out 5.6

Developing self-confidence 1

Recent accomplishments

- What have been your accomplishments over the last few weeks and months? List them and try to recall them in the form of an image of what you did and how it made you feel.
- Why not also set some short-term goals for the next few days and weeks?

Over to Adrian . . .

It became obvious to me in rebuilding my confidence after 1984 that I wasn't able to accept the long-term goal of winning the next Olympics for a while. I needed some quick wins to make me feel good about myself, and the Gold Medal at the Olympics just seemed too far away. At the beginning of the year I set myself a goal to win the British Championships in four months' time, and set a specific time that I thought was within my capability. It was important to get on the first rung of the ladder, out of the mental pit I thought I had sunk into. Right now in business I try as much as possible to break down larger goals and feel good about some of the smaller things that I achieve.

For instance, expanding our business into America is quite a big stretch. Having a market entry plan and a long-term aim is all very well and good for the future direction, but it was vitally important to win some client contracts early on and to build up some good experiences. Just by getting simple feedback from purchase and delivery, we were able to build confidence that our long-term vision was correct.

Drawing on own and others' experiences

Since confidence is largely a function of the situation and circumstances you find yourself in, it can be enhanced in a number of ways via reflecting on your own and others' recent experiences of being in similar situations. The first involves identifying the characteristics of anticipated pressured environments before you encounter them. Who will be involved? How many people will be there? What do you know about them? What will the physical environment be like? Have you performed in the same physical environment before? You may have actually performed in front of the same people in the same physical environment as the upcoming event. If not, you are likely to have performed in environments with similar characteristics on previous occasions.

The key is to identify the things you did well on those previous occasions and the learning points that you will take forward into the upcoming situation. There may be things that you associate with success in those situations, such as preparing in a specific manner or adopting a particular mindset. Think about repeating these things to give your confidence a helping hand.

Another way of enhancing confidence is to reflect on other people and their successes in the context of the performance demands you are about to encounter. Observe them carefully, pick out the things that contributed to their success and focus on enacting them yourself. Role models can be particularly important in this respect. You will have watched and listened to them very carefully over a prolonged period. How do they enhance their confidence in pressured situations? You could even talk to them about it.

Finally, you can create and deal with the pressured situations before you even encounter them physically. A number of years ago I was with a young and very nervous ice skater on the day before the biggest event of his life up to that time. We entered the empty stadium and made our way to the middle of the rink. He surveyed the empty seats all around him and closed his eyes. He imagined the stadium full of spectators and the buzz of excitement as he skated out to the middle of the rink. He imagined himself as being at his most confident and how that had felt on previous occasions. He imagined the music beginning and he skated the whole routine in his head. He took this image away and replayed it several times before the big event. The following evening, the now confident skater won the British Championship.

This is a technique that is very powerful when used in the right manner, and across all types of situation. I have worked with business performers who have rehearsed difficult conversations with their bosses and peers in their heads beforehand. They have identified what they have done well in similar circumstances in the past and used this as a source of confidence in their imagery before the event.

Work through Time-Out 5.7 below to identify how you can enhance your confidence using the techniques described above.

Time-Out 5.7

Developing self-confidence 2

Drawing on own and others' experiences

- Think about some situations in the near future that you know will put you under pressure. Who will be involved? What do you know about them? Have you performed in the same or similar environment or circumstances before? What are the things you did well on those previous occasions?
- What have you observed in other people who deal well with the same or similar circumstances? What can you learn from them?

Over to Adrian . . .

My swimming coach and I discussed another way of building confidence, and that certainly fitted in with one of the approaches Graham describes. Having told him that my long-term goal was to win the Olympics, we identified a current Olympic champion for me to observe at one European competition. I watched the way he warmed up for his race, the way he focused and all his interactions with people. I started to realise that these were simple things that I could do, and I started to imagine myself in his shoes. I created certain routines at future competitions that included my own version of what an Olympic Champion would do.

Managing self-talk

The content of your self-talk reflects your current thoughts in terms of how much confidence you have in a specific situation. Self-talk is usually so automatic that you don't notice it or the effect it has on your moods and feelings. Self-talk that results in low confidence is typically negative and irrational, but almost always sounds like the truth! It's important, therefore, that you slow down and examine the content of your self-talk and how it makes you feel.

Recognising the types of self-talk words you use, together with their impact, can be enlightening. There are three types of self-talk that are prominent in people who are prone to low confidence:[23]

1 **The worrier** – the worrier's dominant tendencies include anticipating the worst, overestimating the odds of something bad or embarrassing happening and creating images of spectacular failure. Typical of the worrier's self-talk is 'what if…?'

2 **The critic** – the critic is that part of you that is constantly judging and evaluating your behaviour. It points out your flaws and limitations and jumps on any mistake you make to remind you that you are a failure. The critic may be personified in your own dialogue as the voice of your mother or father, or anyone in the past who wounded you with their criticism. Typical of the critic's self-talk is 'you stupid…' and 'can't you ever get it right'.

---

[23] Edmund J. Bourne, *The Anxiety and Phobia Workbook*, New Harbinger Publications, Oakland, California, 1995.

3 **The victim** – the victim is that part of you that feels helpless or hopeless and believes that you are in some way deprived, defective or unworthy. The victim always sees insurmountable problems between you and your goals, and bemoans and complains about things as they stand at present. Typical self-talk engaged in by the victim include 'I'll never be able to do that so what's the point in trying' and 'nothing ever goes right'.

The most effective way to deal with negative self-talk is to counter it with positive, supportive statements. This involves writing down and rehearsing positive statements which directly refute or invalidate your negative self-talk, and then to practise using them. There are three rules for using positive self-talk to counter negative thoughts:

- Avoid negatives – instead of saying 'I'm not going to get stressed by this situation', try 'I am confident and calm about this situation'.
- Use the present tense – instead of saying 'I'll be ok in a few minutes', try 'relax and let these feelings pass'.
- Believe in your positive self-talk – do not kid yourself. Only use self-talk that has personal credibility for you.

Negative self-talk reflects the thoughts that are consuming you and causing low confidence. They represent self-limiting mental habits that need to be broken by noticing occasions when you are experiencing them and countering them with positive, rational self-statements. Working through Time-out 5.8 below will help you with this.

Time-Out 5.8

Developing self-confidence 3

Managing self-talk

- Do you talk to yourself in a negative way?
- What are the things you say to yourself?
- How does it affect you?
- What are the positive statements you can say to yourself to counter this negative self-talk?

Over to Adrian . . .

I mentioned earlier in the book that I worked hard on the skill of turning negative self-talk into more positive 'chatter'. The process for me was to build my awareness of those times when I felt I was being negative, and then to really challenge the assumptions I was making. Did I really believe that I had to beat the whole world in this race? There were only seven other competitors! Did I really believe that I would sink and swallow water? No, the last time that happened was when I was 9 years old! I started the process by consciously acting as my own mental sparring partner, and, as previously mentioned, if the negative voice became too loud, I would imagine turning down the volume switch on him, and give the quieter, more positive voice the megaphone.

Interpreting your readiness to perform in a positive way

Think about when you are in a pressured situation and the nerves are jangling. How does this intense response affect your confidence? In my previous life as a researcher into the psychology of elite sport performance, results of our studies consistently showed the very best performers to interpret their intense pre-performance mental and physical response as being facilitative to their performance. They view it as being a sign of their mind and body preparing themselves for the performance ahead. The physical response, in the most obvious forms of muscle tension, sweaty palms and restlessness, is interpreted as the body mobilising itself for the task ahead. The mental response, sometimes in the form of worry, is interpreted as a sign that the event is important and that the performer will give his or her best. In this way, these performers are able to control how they think about what is happening to them under pressure and to use it as a source of confidence.

This process of being able to positively interpret what may be a very intense mental and physical response to pressure involves being able to identify what actually happens to you and then associate it with the upcoming performance demands. Using self-talk to convince yourself that a pounding heart is a positive sign of readiness before difficult meetings may be required in the early stages. The key message is to use your response to pressure in a positive way rather than to fight against it. Try to find ways of achieving this using Time-Out 5.9 below.

Time-Out 5.9

Developing self-confidence 4

Interpreting your readiness to perform in a positive way

- What characterises your mental and physical response prior to an important event, say a presentation, meeting, interview etc?
- How do you interpret these responses?
- How can you change or modify your interpretation to achieve a more positive mindset in the future?

Over to Adrian . . .

Another thing that becomes challenging is when you are about to 'do' a performance, whether it be in business or in sport. In my current role I speak a lot to large groups of people – something that my shy 12 year-old self would have run a mile from in the past. But having been in similar performance situations in sport where I had to stand up and perform, I use the same mindset, i.e. when I feel nervous (mentally or physically) I just know that's what happens naturally before you do something that's important to you. These are all signs that you are getting ready. A sport psychologist once told me that everyone gets butterflies in the stomach when nervous – the trick is to get them to fly in the same formation!

After thinking about these signs of being 'ready', I then start to relax more because it's not something I should be scared of - I've come through it on many occasions, I know I can cope.

A couple of other strategies and techniques

Avoid self-handicapping

Self-handicapping is something that has intrigued me for a considerable time. It is based on the principle that bad luck always seems to strike at the worst possible moment. An executive wakes up with a blinding headache on the morning of a very important meeting. A man on his way to a dream job interview gets stuck in heavy traffic. A runner strains a muscle minutes before a big race. At first sight these would appear to be examples of cruel fate, but research on self-handicapping[24] has unearthed that in many instances such mishaps may be carefully orchestrated

[24] S.Berglas, Self-Handicapping; Etiological and Diagnostic Considerations. In R.L.Higgins, C.R. Snyder & S.Berglas (Eds), *Self-Handicapping. The Paradox That Isn't*, Plenum, 1990.

schemes of the subconscious mind. In other words, people may engage in a form of self-defeating behaviour known as 'self-handicapping', which is essentially a strategy for conveniently explaining under-performance.

Psychologists refer to the 'Deschapelles coup' to reflect acts of self-sabotage amongst performers. Deschapelles was an 18th century French chess player who quickly became a champion, but as the competition grew stronger he adopted a new condition for all matches; he would only compete if his opponent would remove one of Deschapelles' pawns and make the first move. Since this increased the odds of him losing, he could blame any loss on his opponent's advantage, but if he won then he would become revered for his amazing skills. Taking on a handicap allows performers to save face when failure does occur, but it also impacts upon confidence because the odds of succeeding are reduced. The people most likely to be self-handicappers are performers who are obsessed with success – they need a pre-prepared 'excuse' for when they do not succeed.

Think back to some previous performances and things that have threatened your performance beforehand – headaches, mysterious ailments, unforeseen circumstances, etc. Is there a regular pattern? Remember that it is a strategy used before you perform rather than after it, and also that it is often subconscious. The key to dealing with self-handicapping is identifying if and how you do it. Try to rule it out of any equation in predicting how you perform – you may find that such unfortunate circumstances become less frequent and that confidence is enhanced.

When blaming everything else is allowed

My work as a sport psychologist has been characterised by working with fascinating people who have fascinating ways of maintaining confidence in the most pressured situations. A few years ago I was helping an English cricket batsman understand how he remained confident under pressure for the purpose of writing about it in his biography. He was well known amongst his peers for his supreme confidence at the wicket, but his relative lack of confidence off the field. He told me that early in an innings when he sometimes felt out of form, he would attribute his 'playing and missing' or lack of timing to anything other than *him* – the superb quality of the bowling, the unpredictable nature of the wicket, etc. His poor form was nothing to do with him and so his confidence could remain high. When he was eventually dismissed he would analyse his performance in the minutest detail and work out what he was doing wrong and therefore needed to work on. He would often then go to the practice nets and work on those aspects of his batting until he thought he had resolved the problem.

What the cricketer was doing while he was performing at the wicket was attributing his failure to external factors in the environment – things he could not control so that they need not dent his confidence. This is known in psychology as a 'self-serving bias' where inaccurate attributions are made to protect a performer's confidence in the moment. This is effective and allowable *only* when performers then reflect on their performance after the event and check that they were accurate attributions. Where, in fact, the reasons for failure are internal to the performer, then working on these aspects of performance and improving them can also help to build confidence.

Where do you start?

Self-confidence is different from self-esteem – you can do something about it almost immediately. Pay particular attention to the images you conjure up and the self-talk you engage in when under pressure because they are likely to have a big impact on your level of confidence. Try experimenting with the techniques and strategies described in this section and find out what works for you.

Chris Andy Scott Emma Studies

Chris

The pressure had got to Chris to the extent that he had lost sight of what a good coach he was. The solution was actually relatively straightforward; he needed to remind himself of his achievements as a coach and the accolades he had received throughout his career. He concentrated on his tangible and non-tangible achievements, and what they provided evidence of and what they were underpinned by respectively. Chris quickly recalled that the successes of the teams he had coached were due to more than just the ability and skills of the individual players; they were also the result of a long list of his own abilities and skills that included being innovative, analytical and making difficult decisions under pressure. He had done it before and he knew he could do it again.

Andy

Andy's situation was a classic example of letting the environment and other people determine his self-confidence. This was exacerbated by the fact that his self-esteem was relatively low. This is where he started. He revisited his assertions that he had been lucky to reach his current position. He recognised that he was attributing his success to external factors, and began to rationalise how his own ability, skills and talents had been important contributors to his achievements. The internal and constant nature of these factors meant that he had been ignoring crucial ▶

personal attributes that could form the foundation of his self-esteem. Andy wrote the factors on a card that he would carry in a wallet as a constant reminder. He also identified his very high expectations of himself as something he could never live up to. He identified a perfectionist tendency that meant he was never satisfied with his performance. Accepting fallibility and being more realistic about what was possible proved to be an effective means of challenging his expectations and building his self-esteem.

Scott

Scott's self-belief was shattered by his continual 'failures' during the season to date. But his short-term needs superseded everything else. He worked on his confidence prior to and during tournaments. His self-talk emerged as a key factor because it was mainly around telling himself things like 'I'm not good enough to compete at this level' and 'I can't afford to mess up today'.

Scott realised that such self-statements were extremely unhelpful and set about developing positive statements to counter them; 'I'm confident that I can compete well at this level' and 'Today is an opportunity to show what I can do'. He also worked on his interpretation of his physical and mental state immediately prior to and early in competitive rounds. He had grown to hate the mental anxiety and physical tension he felt in the lead-up to a tournament. The relaxation Scott had learned (see Chapter 4) helped calm these symptoms to manageable proportions, but he also needed a way of thinking of them as helping his preparation. He began to see it as a natural part of the pre-performance process and that it was a sign that his mind and body were readying themselves for performing at their best. Scott's management of his self-talk and the way he thought about his pre-performance nerves were a big factor in his subsequent increase in self-confidence prior to tournaments.

Emma

Emma's belief in herself was not as robust as she thought. Her need to prove herself to her male colleagues reflected a self-belief that was not fully internalised – she was relying on their approval and recognition as an acceptance of her competence. And Emma's need to demonstrate her abilities and skills resulted in an inflexibility that damaged working relations with the very people she needed reinforcement from. She refused to budge on decisions, and was reluctant to listen to and consider others' views. Emma started working on instilling a deeper internalisation of her self-esteem by recognising that her behaviour with her male colleagues was founded on her concerns for how others perceived her. She was able to see how this resulted in self-handicapping – she was an undervalued female at the mercy of her male colleagues! She moved forward by beginning to think of herself as a performer rather than as a woman. Emma worked out that she had achieved her senior position as a function of her performance. The fact that she was a woman was irrelevant!

In a nutshell

- Self-belief comprises two key components - self-esteem and self-confidence.
- Self-esteem is a way of thinking and feeling that implies that you accept, respect and trust yourself.
- Self-esteem is a function of how you typically attribute success and failure and how you think about your achievements in life.
- Self-confidence reflects your optimism about being successful in specific situations and circumstances.
- Self-confidence is a function of recent performance accomplishments, drawing on your own and others' experiences, managing self-talk and how you interpret your mental and physical response under pressure.

What next?

- Recognise how you typically attribute success and failure and the impact this has on your self-esteem.
- Understand the abilities, beliefs and values that lie at the core of you and then take pride in them.
- Let go of any perfectionist tendencies that cause problems for you.
- Experiment with the various strategies and techniques for enhancing self-confidence.
- Learn to recognise when you are engaging in self-defeating, self-handicapping thoughts and behaviours, and then stop engaging in them!

6 Making Your Motivation Work for You

After reading this chapter you will know about:

- How to motivate yourself to optimum levels
- How to recover from setbacks
- How to set INSPIRED goals

Skills and abilities alone will not deliver high performance that is sustainable. Motivation is the key to directing and guiding those skills and abilities to their best possible effect. But it is not simply a case of being motivated. Motivation can assume many forms, and not all of them are conducive to high performance, at least not at a sustainable level. This chapter examines and describes how you can achieve optimum motivation so that it works *for* rather than *against* you.

→ How far are you prepared to go to achieve your ambitions?

One thing is for sure amongst the very best performers; they are all very highly motivated individuals. Sometimes, people's motivation can be so great that they go to extraordinary lengths to achieve their ambitions. A senior executive in a global organisation achieved legendary status for the lengths he would go to in pursuing his aspirations to get to the top. Based in the US, he faced the dilemma of having to attend an important three-day meeting in London which meant that he would miss a dinner in New York where he would be sitting at the table of the most senior and influential figures in the organisation. Such was the intensity of his burning ambition that the solution was actually quite simple; at the end of the first day of the meeting in London he flew back for the dinner, spending five hours in New York before returning on an overnight flight to London for the 8.30 start on the second day.

Such stories are familiar amongst performers who at times can seem obsessed with success. It became clear to me that a top ten world-ranked performer was using the meditative relaxation technique we had worked on to distract her from an injury that troubled her during competitive matches. Her desire to become Number One was so great that she prioritised it above her own well-being. But this should be no real surprise – remember the US study described in Chapter 2 which revealed that 52% of world-class athletes surveyed would take a drug that would make them unbeatable for the next five years even though they knew they would die afterwards.

The pressure that performers like those referred to above impose on themselves is enormous, and there is a seemingly 'unhealthy' aspect to their motives. They are willing to make huge sacrifices to achieve their ambitions. The very best performers I have worked with do not see themselves as making 'sacrifices' because this is not a good foundation for their motivation. Instead, they are careful to emphasise the 'choices' they have made. If they viewed the time they spent in a gruelling training environment, or on a plane travelling to meeting after meeting and being away from loved ones as a sacrifice, then their longer-term motivation would be in jeopardy.

These people are capable of extraordinary commitment because they have *chosen* to do so and know how far to take it; it is not something that they *must* do at any cost. Theirs is a 'healthy' motivation that forms a crucial element in enabling them to bounce back from setbacks and disappointments because they are able to rationalise and put things in perspective. They use setbacks as part of their continued development, rather than seeing them as disasters that threaten their aspirations.

→ So what's next?

Motivation is not just a constant, day-to-day drive towards achieving carefully-considered goals. At the risk of getting overly philosophical, it is about your very existence and what you stand for; it is your reason for being. It is important, therefore, to take regular time-outs to reflect on and examine what is driving you and why, and to modify the foundations of your motives if necessary.

A classic case in point is what happens when you have achieved *the* ambition that you have focused on for so long? I have come across a number of people who have achieved what they thought was their 'life-time goal' – performers who have won that Olympic Gold Medal or World Championship, entrepreneurs who have built a company and have made their millions through a sale, executives who have achieved that managing director status. These performers have been highly achievement-driven for most or all of their lives and reach a point where they find themselves with no other obvious achievements to aim for. Some people do not cope very well with these circumstances. They may begin to question the meaning of life and actually become quite unhappy because they perceive themselves to have no direction any more.

Others deal with this situation in a much more constructive manner by 'transferring' their motivation to other things. Adrian did just that, as he describes in his section below.

Over to Adrian . . .

Having won my Olympic Gold Medal in 1988 at the age of 23, I continued my swimming career up to the next Olympics where I finally retired at the relatively old age (in those days!) for swimmers of 27. I continued my career beyond 1988 because I knew that there were still even better performances in me, so I followed the path of continuous development. When I finished eighth in the final in the 1992 Barcelona Olympics, I knew that my best was now not good enough and that there was no more to extract from myself. It was time to retire.

After I retired, I did feel a bit lost. Nothing could prepare me for the change that came my way, however much I had thought and planned beforehand. It was obvious that swimming fast was not going to be much use in the business world, so I had to reflect on other skills and qualities that I had. It was really important for me to find a career that had a future focus, that would stretch me, not just in achievement terms but to develop me as a person. I knew that once I found my 'thing' that I would be motivated to achieve the best I could. I had also realised quite soon afterwards that, at my best, I was focused on one career, swimming; I just had to find the next career and work hard at it. There were obvious challenges, not least the fact that I had performed as an individual in swimming, whereas in business I was going to have to be a lot more 'user friendly'!

▶

> **Working on how to communicate my goals and what I am thinking is a great challenge for me still, because I know that these goals may switch *me* on, but I need to help find what motivates *others* and try to match them with our company goals.**

There are other, better known stories of high achievers who are constantly seeking other, more personal challenges in other spheres of performance. Such high-profile individuals include Sir Richard Branson whose exploits and adventures outside the business world have been well documented in recent years. Attempts at achieving world records in hot air balloons and the like are the sign of an individual on a paradoxical never-ending journey of self-fulfilment. Explorer Sir Ranulf Fiennes, who ran seven marathons on seven different continents in seven days, provides an extraordinary example of people who require constant personal challenges. Another aspect to the motivation of such people is that their achievements are often tied into good causes, such as charities. In this way they are benefiting society, which can provide them with another sense of achievement.

Some key questions about motivation

Motivation is a fundamental driving force behind people's behaviour and performance. It should be no surprise to learn, therefore, that there is a huge scientific literature and tons of popular psychology books on the topic. Thus, knowing where to start in getting to grips with motivation is no easy task. This section addresses a series of basic questions that will help you understand the foundations of your own motivation.

Are you motivated for the right reasons?

Behaviour, at the most basic level, can be broken down into two very different types: 'approach' and 'avoidance' behaviours. **Approach** behaviour is where you quite literally approach or move toward some set of circumstances; **avoidanc**e behaviour, on the other hand, is where you avoid or move away from a set of circumstances. These behaviours are underpinned and driven by 'approach' and 'avoidance motivation' respectively.

In my one-to-one coaching of senior executives I have sometimes come across individuals who tell me that 'it's time to move on so I've decided to look for another job'. Classic approach motives include recognising that they have developed and learned as much as they can in their current environment and need new circumstances in which they can continue to develop. They may wish to stretch themselves further by the challenge of a new role in a different type of organisation, or it may be the next natural step to achieving their career ambitions. They have very positive reasons for leaving and have mapped out their future.

Those executives who are driven by avoidance motives, on the other hand, often refer to being worn down by frustrations in their current role, the people they work with, or perhaps the lack of vision in the organisation. They are often fed up and disillusioned and want to get away at the earliest opportunity. They have the impression that things will be different elsewhere, but may not be sure what they want to move to – their main motive is to avoid their current set of circumstances. These are not the best motives for leaving and these people sometimes find themselves in other jobs that they find equally or even more disappointing. They have, in effect, spent too much time looking back and not enough time focusing on the future.

In sport it is common to read about performers who are driven mainly by the fear of failing. This is a very strong motivator for some performers, but think about the anguish that they experience prior to important events and the desperation they feel following failure. For some performers it may be that they are not willing to put themselves in situations in which they might fail – a classic avoidance behaviour. In my experience the very best performers are driven more by the desire for success, an approach motive which means that they look forward to important competitions and take time to learn from their failures.

Over to Adrian . . .

I won the Olympics at my second attempt in 1998 at the age of 24, and I spent some time coming to terms with the fact that I had achieved the main dream that I had been carrying for 12 years. A number of people suggested that I 'quit at the top'. I didn't, and carried on for a further four years. I needed to make sure that I had squeezed as much out of my swimming talent as possible. I had some great years, and indeed some of my most successful ones.

However, when it came to retiring I was in no doubt that I had to move on. I was actually looking forward to my life outside sport. It was very daunting, and certainly not easy, but I am sure that I had committed to an *approach* motive, in that I never for one minute considered going back to swimming. I see a lot of sports people announce their retirement, but soon afterwards make (in the main) much-regretted comebacks. It seems to me that they have not created the future view, and often find it too frustrating to start a new career, so they go back to sport, probably as an *avoidance* motive for anything that they perceive won't match up to their experiences in sport.

What is the main driver of *your* motivation? You will probably need to think about your day-to-day motivation as well as your longer-term goals to get a good feel for how you might approach or avoid particular sets of circumstances. Excessive pressure that is experienced as stress can drive avoidance motivation so reflect, in particular, on how your motives might change as a function of being under stress.

Are there times when you just do not give a damn?

A number of years ago a series of experiments conducted with laboratory dogs revealed some fascinating findings that are readily applicable to human beings.[25] The experiments involved administering shocks to three dogs in different conditions. The first dog was able to turn off the shock by pushing a panel with its nose. The second dog was given exactly the same shocks as the first, but had no means of escaping them. The third dog received no shocks at all. Following this experience, the dogs were placed in a box with two compartments that were separated by a low barrier. When administered the shocks, all the dogs had to do to escape them was to jump over the barrier from one compartment to the other. Within seconds the first dog that had been taught that it could control the shocks discovered that it could jump over the barrier to escape them, as did the third dog that had received no shocks at all. The second dog that had found that nothing that it did mattered, made no effort to escape – it lay down even though it continued to receive shocks. This dog never discovered that it could escape the shocks by simply jumping over a small barrier.

[25] Source: Martin Seligman, *Learned Optimism: How To Change Your Mind and Your Life*, Pocket Books, 1998.

The second dog was experiencing 'learned helplessness' – it had learned that nothing it did could make a difference to the circumstances it found itself in, so why try! Hopefully, you have never suffered from learned helplessness, but there may have been times when you have felt like giving up because nothing you do seems to make any difference. So why bother and why care? Perhaps the closest thing to learned helplessness amongst most sport and business performers is the experience of burnout. One of the classic symptoms of burnout is not caring, 'not giving a damn anymore'. Disengagement, apathy, acquiescence and passiveness are all behaviours and attitudes associated with this apparent lack of motivation. It is an unpleasant and sometimes destructive state to be in. Watch out for early signs!

Over to Adrian . . .

As someone preparing and racing to be the best in the world, there was no way I could ever entertain the thought that I could not make a difference. On reflection I think that I had a good group of friends and family who would support and encourage me to change the situation if I was not happy. In work I think it is important to find those people who give you energy, rather than take it from you. In those early stages of 'burnout', the last thing you need is your closest friend or work colleague agreeing with your negative thoughts.

How important are *you* in your motivation?

Who is the most important person in the world to you? I have asked this question of sport and business performers on numerous occasions over the years and the answer I receive is almost always someone other than themselves – 'my wife', 'my boyfriend', 'my child'. Further questioning leads them to the conclusion that it is, in fact, *themselves*, and that important others can only be happy when they themselves are happy. This stimulates them to reflect on their own needs and to find ways of satisfying them.

I have come across a number of performers whose motives are sometimes excessively focused on others' needs. Some of the younger sport performers I have worked with have found themselves in a sport because their parents have been keen for them to take part, and in some cases have funded their participation to quite extreme levels. These performers are very aware of their parents' desires for their success and have been 'doing it for them' rather than to satisfy their own needs. This does not bode well for long-term participation or even enjoyment.

Although not as prevalent in business, I have encountered some performers who have been working hard to satisfy the needs of important others, maybe that partner who wants to retire to that big house in the country, or those children who need an expensive education. At the extreme of putting others' needs before your own is something known as a 'subjugation schema'. This manifests in things like:

- not liking to disagree with others' opinions;
- worrying about doing and saying things that might hurt others' feelings;
- staying in situations where you are trapped or where your needs are not met;
- not wanting to appear selfish so that you go to the other extreme;
- not knowing what you want or prefer in many situations;
- often sacrificing yourself for the sake of others;
- standing up for other people's rights when they are in trouble;
- being weak in negotiations;
- not asking for promotions or salary increases at work;
- playing down your accomplishments.

The key to ensuring the importance of satisfying your own needs is twofold. Firstly, you should recognise your own well-being as being important in determining the well-being of people who are particularly important and close to you. Secondly, there is an obvious risk of becoming or appearing selfish in putting your own needs first. This requires a fine balancing act in terms of focusing on your own needs and weighing up the extent to which you can also satisfy others' needs. Remember this key message – do it for yourself, not for other people!

Over to Adrian . . .

I think that I upset a number of people during my swimming career by being just a little bit too self-centred. I was very determined to achieve success for myself, that nothing, or nobody was going to get in the way; not exactly a 'subjugation schema'! However, in moving into business, I have become quite aware of my strengths and many weaknesses. On the one hand, I do encourage people to look inside themselves to find what they are passionate about, and try to bring that to the job. On the other hand, I also find myself overcompensating for my past selfishness. It sometimes feels as though I have subjugated my own identity into that of the company. It seems strange, but occasionally, I have to remind myself to keep an eye on my own aspirations.

Do you enjoy your motivation?

This may seem a bizarre question at first sight, but for some performers the achievement of their goals and ambitions means so much to them that they are unable to enjoy the journey. For these performers, motivation and self-imposed pressure are often the same thing. When goals are not achieved they can experience quite intense symptoms of stress, that debilitating side of pressure that exacerbates the downward spiral that sometimes ensues. At the extreme, negative motivation can manifest in an obsession with and desperation for success, with anything less being an abject failure. Motivation in this form can be a far from enjoyable experience.

For those performers who are 'positively motivated' the experience is a very different one. Their goals are challenging, but always realistic, ensuring that they are continually stretching themselves, but not to ridiculous limits. Their goals are the result of careful reflection of what they are capable of and are broken down into shorter-term goals that give them a sense of achievement and satisfaction as they progress. Their motivation is manifested in an energy and exhilaration that drives them to continuous improvement, but which allows them to stop occasionally to 'smell the roses along the way'.

How much do you 'enjoy' your own motivation? Do you go to bed at night and wake up the next morning looking forward to the challenges of the day ahead? Or do you lie awake at night worrying about the threats to your ambitions that you will encounter the following day?

Over to Adrian . . .

I think that I have worked this one out for myself, but it has taken me a long time! I spent so long in swimming just looking for the next mountain to climb (or medal to win!) that I forgot to take in the view. I remember reading a newspaper article about a race I had swum, in which I had equalled my own World Record, and the journalist said that I looked like the unhappiest person in the pool. It's great when other people give you these gems of feedback! Luckily, I read this one and decided to do something about it. Even then, it wasn't until a few years after I had retired from swimming that I actually 'allowed' myself to think good things about my career.

Where is your motivation focused?

You may have heard the following story, or a version of it, but I will remind you of it anyway because it emphasises a very important aspect of motivation.

There was an old man who moved into a house with a brick wall surrounding it. One day, a group of kids began playing football outside the old man's house, using his wall as one of their goals. The noise of the ball striking the wall was loud and continuous and disrupted the old man's peace and quiet that he so longed for. The old man went out to the kids and asked them to play further down the street. One of the kids responded, 'sorry but we've been playing football here after school for a long time now. Your wall provides us with a perfect goal and we really enjoy playing here.' The old man thought for a few moments and then asked, 'if I give you each 25p will you please go and play somewhere else?' The kids reluctantly agreed and the old man went inside to resume his afternoon rest.

The following afternoon at the same time, the old man again heard the ball thudding against his wall. He went outside and again offered the kids 25p to play somewhere else. They refused, reiterating that they derived particular pleasure from playing in that location because the wall provided such a good goal. The old man then offered them 50p each to play somewhere else and they reluctantly agreed to move on. The following day at the same time the old man was yet again woken by the noise of the kids playing football outside his house. He went outside and this time had to pay them 75p each to move on from the place where they so enjoyed playing after school.

The following day the kids were yet again playing football outside the old man's house, but this time he failed to appear. The kids went to his door and knocked on it. The old man appeared and the kids said, 'we're playing football outside your house. Why have you not come out and paid us to move on?' The old man replied, 'I can't. I have no money left to pay you.' The kids then retorted, 'if that's the case, there's no point in playing outside your house. We'll play somewhere else.'

This story reflects a basic distinction that has been around for a long time in the research and popular psychology literature between 'internal' and 'external' motivation. It also shows how the nature of motivation can change as a function of the performance environment and the rewards that are on offer. The kids were originally motivated internally by the pleasure they derived from playing football against the old man's wall that provided such a perfect goal. However, this internal motivation was slowly eroded and eventually destroyed by the gradually increasing external motivation the old man provided in the form of payment to play somewhere else. So when the old man had run out of money to pay them, there was no internal motivation remaining. They were no longer playing for enjoyment; they were playing for money.

I was asked some time ago to work with a young, very talented international team sport performer whose performance had dropped off worryingly over the past few months. He had achieved international level at an early age, and his personality and marketability meant that he was bound to attract media attention outside the back pages of the tabloids. He was in demand in a big way and his focus was as much, if not even more, on his earning potential as a celebrity than on his continuous development as a sport performer. Here was a classic case of a young kid enjoying a sport he was very good at, being thrust into an environment where he got paid for playing his sport and other, very lucrative external rewards were in abundance. But in this case, they had taken over his motivation.

This type of situation is prevalent in business where the assumption tends to be that it is the external rewards that will drive performance. They often do, of course, but the problem is that it is often to the detriment of internal motivation. Organisations that provide their performers with substantial bonuses for hitting performance targets essentially control their motivation. For performers who are externally motivated over prolonged periods, their internal motivation subsides so that they become heavily dependent on the material rewards to keep going. Another important aspect of external motivation is that it can drive quite extreme behaviours in the quest for those rewards, often resulting in stress and burn-out.

Where is *your* motivation focused? Is it internally-focused around achievement for your own pride, enjoyment, interest and satisfaction, or is it more the external rewards and incentives that you are enticed by? This is a very important dimension of motivation that is explored in greater depth in the following section.

Over to Adrian . . .

After I made the British swimming team, and then started to win international races, I spent about a week getting frustrated and upset that we didn't get paid in swimming – 'just look at those footballers – if only I was one of them'. Luckily, I had just about the most grounded set of parents and friends anyone could hope to have. At dinner one evening, I had barely got one of my whinges out, when I had a barrage of abuse back. 'Well you're not, so just get on with it. You are one of the luckiest people alive, being able to find a talent for something, and you are representing the country . . .' As I say, it didn't take long to remember why I was doing it!

What is the essence of *your* motivation?

You have been posed five important questions in this section that will help you to better understand the key drivers of your motivation, and whether it works for or against you. Record your reflections in Time-Out 6.1.

Time-Out 6.1

Capturing the essence of your motivation

Are you motivated for the right reasons?
What is the main driver of your motivation? You will probably need to think about your day-to-day motivation as well as your longer-term goals to get a good feel for how you might *approach* or *avoid* particular sets of circumstances. Excessive pressure that is experienced as stress can drive avoidance motivation so reflect, in particular, on how your motives might change as a function of being under stress.

Are there times when you just do not give a damn?
Are there times when you stop caring and don't give a damn anymore? Do you disengage from people and/or situations? What do you associate with these times?

How important are *you* in your motivation?
Do you focus excessively on others' needs and put them before your own? Do you refrain from disagreeing with others' opinions in case you hurt their feelings? Do you stay in situations where you feel trapped or where your needs are not met?

Do you enjoy your motivation?
How much do you 'enjoy' your own motivation? Do you go to bed at night and wake up the next morning looking forward to the challenges of the day ahead? Or do you lie awake at night worrying about the threats to your ambitions that you will encounter the following day?

Where is your motivation focused?
Where is your motivation focused? Is it internally-focused around achievement for your own pride, enjoyment, interest and satisfaction, or is it more the external rewards and incentives that you are enticed by?

→ A closer look at internal and external motivation

My experience as one of the psychologists to the Great Britain Olympic team in 1996 left me with many rich and unforgettable memories, and also with the odd bizarre one. I can recall one particular incident vividly because it was such a surprise to me. It began when I was having breakfast with members of the team a couple of weeks before the Games were to be opened. Chatting to a performer, Sandra, who was eagerly awaiting the arrival of her coach from England, the conversation meandered into her training plan for the day and how she was waiting for the day's training schedule to be faxed through from the coach. I wished her well and set off on my own schedule for the day. At the end of a gruelling day's training for the athletes in the heat and humidity, I passed Sandra in the corridor and was surprised at her remarkably fresh appearance. My enquiry about how her training had gone that day was met with the reply 'I didn't train. The fax didn't arrive.'

I was astonished. Here was an elite performer just about to enter the biggest sporting arena of her life who had missed a valuable opportunity to train. Sandra had sat around the athletes' lounge for most of the day waiting for a fax that would never arrive. It would be natural to wonder why she did not take matters into her own hands and at least improvise with an impromptu training session. As it was, she missed out on the vital opportunity of a day's acclimatisation to performing in the intense heat and humidity.

Sandra's motivation and behaviour puzzled me greatly because both seemed to be determined by her coach. My experience had been that the very best performers' behaviours at this level, even in lucratively rewarded sports, are determined mainly by internal motivation. They are unable to put in the long, often gruelling training sessions without the strong foundation of internal motivation, but here was what seemed to be a very significant element of external motivation and dependence in this particular performer.

This story demonstrates that the basic distinction between internal and external motivation, whilst very important, is too simple to explain many aspects of behaviour and that motivation needs to be broken down further in order to better understand its more complex effects and, most importantly, how to determine and optimise its impact. This section therefore considers several distinct types of motivation and their consequences for performance.

The nature of motivation

Warning: you might find this section hard-going!

Motivation is a particularly complex dimension of the human existence and it is not my intention to baffle you with the intricate details of central issues involved in understanding it and how it determines behaviour. However, it is important to get to grips with some essential elements of what motivation is and how it can have different drivers. You might find the next couple of pages hard-going, but be mentally tough and stick with it!

Let's begin briefly with the basic distinction between internal and external motivation because it is so fundamental in explaining behaviour. Essentially, external-motivation refers to the performance of an activity in order to attain some separable outcome; for example, performing for incentives such as money. Internal motivation, on the other hand, refers to doing an activity for the inherent satisfaction of the activity itself or, in other words, performing simply because you enjoy it. Comparisons between performers whose motivation is internal and those who are externally-motivated or 'controlled' reveal crucial differences that have very significant implications for both well-being and performance.

Research[26] has shown that a strong relative emphasis and focus on the attainment of internal aspirations such as personal growth and development is associated with higher self-esteem, self-actualisation, and lower depression and anxiety. On the other hand, placing strong relative emphasis and focus on external aspirations such as wealth and fame is associated with lower self-esteem and self-actualisation, and higher depression and anxiety. However, it is not merely the 'focus' on internal and external aspirations that is important; the attainment of these different aspirations have essentially the same effects on well-being. Most importantly, internally-motivated performers, when compared to externally-motivated performers, have more interest, excitement and confidence, which in turn leads to greater persistence, creativity, energy, well-being and, crucially, performance. So let's look closer at internal motivation.

Internal motivation

Michael Johnson, the American five-times Olympic Gold Medallist who became the first sprinter in the history of the Olympics to win the 200 and 400 metre events at the same Games, summed up the importance of internal motivation in his advice for others as follows:

> *My best motivation has always come from the pure joy of running and competing, from the same thrill I got as a 10 year-old. Have you ever known a 10 year-old to burn out? Find your initial motivation, the reason you became an architect. That's the secret to persevering.* [27]

Internal motivation is reflected in the value placed on personal growth and development, and the desire to seek out novelty and challenges, to extend and exercise one's capacities, to explore and to learn. As such, it represents a major source of energy and enjoyment that is open to all people. However, for internal motivation to be maintained and enhanced, it is necessary to satisfy three innate psychological needs that apply to people in virtually every domain of life and that are essential for health and well-being:

- competence – a feeling of mastery or accomplishment;
- autonomy – a sense of being in control so that behaviour is self-determined;
- relatedness – a sense of belonging and security.

26 Richard Ryan & Edward Deci, Self-determination theory and the facilitation of intrinsic motivation, social development and well-being, *American Psychologist*, 2000, pp. 68–78

27 Michael Johnson, *Slaying the Dragon*, Harper Collins, 1996, p. 165.

Research[28] has shown that the satisfaction of these needs at work is associated with more positive well-being and higher performance than when they are not experienced. The fluctuation of the satisfaction of these needs on a daily basis also predicts mood, vitality and self-esteem. In sport, internal motivation results in more enjoyment, less pressure and more effort than externally-derived motivation, thus enabling performers to put in the long hours, dedication and commitment to training.

So internal motivation is pretty important to any performer! But there are a number of threats to internal motivation that all performers need to be aware of, including:

- perceiving feedback that is not totally positive as indicating a lack of competence;
- over-valuing tangible rewards so that they become the major driver for good performance;
- being constantly driven by deadlines, directives and imposed goals;
- being unable to establish a secure relational base or sense of attachment to something or someone (although internally-motivated behaviours are often performed in isolation, suggesting that a sense of belonging to someone or something close to you may not be necessary).

There are, therefore, numerous reasons to develop some form of internal motivation for your day-to-day activities. In summary, if your performance is to be maintained and enhanced through internal motivation, it is important that you:

- find ways of feeling competent in what you do;
- are able to exercise choice over your behaviour;
- can relate in some positive way to the people you are performing with or the cause you are contributing to.

Deriving some internal motivation from external motivation

Unfortunately, much of what you do is not internally-motivated. Not everything consumes you with the interest, enjoyment and energy that you would ideally derive. You find yourself in situations carrying out

28 Marylene Gagne & Edward Deci, Self-determination theory and work motivation, *Journal of Organizational Behaviour*, 2005, pp. 331–362.

activities that you would not necessarily choose to be doing if you had complete control – completing those monthly expense forms, attending those meetings with demanding and difficult clients, etc. So how do you motivate yourself for such activities? This is where viewing external motivation as a single entity and merely the opposite of internal motivation is unhelpful. It is simply not as simple as that!

Think about times when you have wanted to alter behaviour in others; perhaps as a leader or manager who wants individuals to work better together as a team, or perhaps as someone who has required greater support from your line manager. Others' motivation to behave in the desired manner can range from unwillingness to passive compliance to active personal commitment. And so, obviously, can yours! These are all different ways of responding to external efforts to alter behaviour and reflect the fact that externally-motivated behaviour varies in its degree of self-determination, or how much control you have over the regulation of that behaviour.

Thus, behaviour is best thought of as varying along a continuum of behavioural regulation that reflects these varying degrees of self-determination. Figure 6.1 (based on the recent work of Richard Ryan and Edward L. Deci[29]) shows how this continuum ranges from 'complete non-self-determined behaviour' at one extreme to 'complete self-determined behaviour' at the other; these represent 'pure external motivation' and 'pure internal motivation' respectively. In between these extremes are the varying degrees of external motivation and self-determined behaviours that become more autonomous as they move towards pure internal motivation. These different levels of self-determined behaviour reflect differing degrees to which you internalise and value the need to behave in a certain way, so that it becomes integrated and transformed into some sense of self-motivation. Like it or not, you will find yourself in situations where certain behaviours and values are prescribed, so that you may need to make an effort to internalise and integrate them to have a sense of self-determination.

29 Richard M Ryan and Edward L Deci, Self Determination Theory and the Facilitation of Intrinsic Motivation, Social Development and Well Being, *American Psychologist*, January 2000, Vol. 55, No. 1, 68–78.

Figure 6.1 To what extent do you determine your motivation and behaviour?

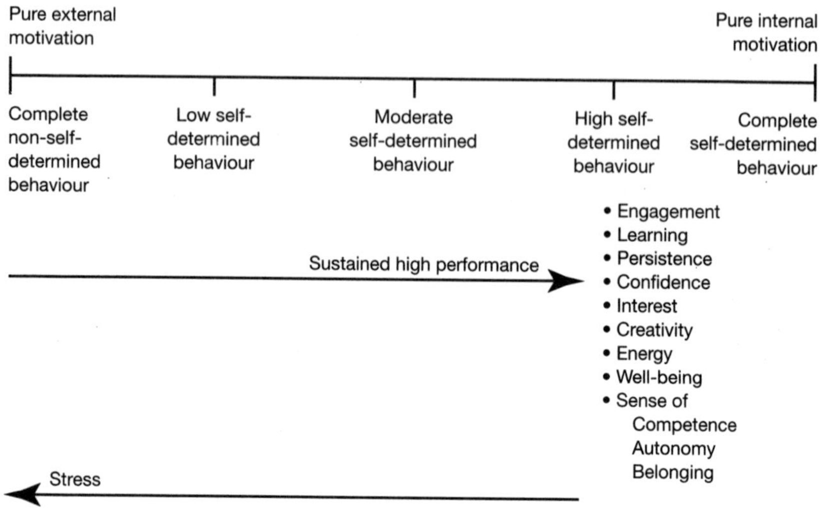

For example, as a leader or manager you may be required to carry out formal, very detailed performance reviews with direct reports. This is complete non-self-determined behaviour if you have no choice nor interest at all in doing them. Approached in this way, performance reviews constitute an obstacle to spending time doing the things that stimulate you. So how do you motivate yourself to carry out the reviews in circumstances where you feel you are being motivated or even controlled by external forces? Devoting time to reflect on the value of performance reviews and identifying the benefits they bring to you and your team or part of the business allows them to take on a different meaning. This is the beginning of the process of internalising and valuing the need so that you are able to derive a sense of self-motivation to conduct performance reviews with the effort and commitment they deserve.

Apply the same principle to, say, a forward in football who may resent that compulsory extra, unexpected Sunday morning training session imposed by the coach following a 5-3 defeat the previous day. Why does he, a forward who scored two goals the day before, need to be at a session targeted at an appalling defence that yielded five goals? This is the last thing he wants or thinks is warranted for him as an individual. Recognising the value of dealing with defensive frailties as a whole team, and offering support and encouragement as part of a 'we're all in it together' mindset will allow him to internalise the need and to generate a sense of self-motivation that will ensure appropriate energy and effort in such circumstances.

The examples above are essentially about being able to self-regulate behaviours in response to external motivation that you do not find internally interesting or necessary, via transforming regulation by external contingencies into regulation by internal ones.

The key to performing optimally when your motivation is externally-driven is to first recognise where along the continuum your motivation lies, and how much autonomy and self-determination of your behaviour you possess. Read through the following and try to get a sense of where your motivation generally lies, and also where it lies for specific activities you carry out on a day-to-day basis.

- **Complete non-self-determined behaviour** – you work hard because you *must*; your motivation is purely external. You conform to required behaviours because you effectively have no choice. It may be because this provides you with the only means of achieving the success that will result in the tangible rewards you must have to live a particular lifestyle. The rewards are likely to be the only things that matter to you in your working life.
- **Low self-determined behaviour** – you work hard because you *need* the rewards you receive for being successful. External recognition may represent a means via which you can feel good about yourself because you equate your personal worth or self-esteem with material symbols of your success – they demonstrate your ability to yourself, but also to others. The need to obtain the rewards is often derived from a need to avoid feeling the guilt or anxiety that can accompany a sense of being a failure. This need is so great that you have little choice but to behave in ways that will satisfy it by striving for external recognition.
- **Moderate self-determined behaviour** – you work hard because you *like* the tangible rewards you receive for success. But they are important to you because they also allow you to do things outside work that you like doing, thus helping to provide a balanced existence. The behaviours that you exhibit to achieve rewards are therefore linked to values that you personally endorse and are thus internalised and integrated in a way that provides a sense of self-determination.
- **High self-determined behaviour** – you work hard because you *enjoy* it. Being successful gives you a sense of personal pride and satisfaction, and the rewards you receive allow you to do things outside work that

you also really enjoy. In this way any external regulations are fully assimilated to the self, which means that they have been evaluated and brought into congruence with your other values and needs.

- **Complete self-determined behaviour** – you work hard solely because you *love* it – this represents motivation that is purely internal. The process of taking part and the enjoyment and interest that you derive from it are all that matter to you. In this way, your behaviours and values are fully internalised and integrated.

Where are you on this continuum most of the time? Where you lie will have a big influence on your ability to deliver sustained high performance. Our research on mental toughness showed two key factors specific to motivation: the ability to bounce back from performance setbacks as a result of increased determination to succeed; and internalised motivation to succeed. The further over to the left you are on the continuum shown in Figure 6.1, the more pressure and stress there is to perform, and the harder it is to recover from setbacks. Furthermore, there is little or no internalised motivation to succeed. Mental toughness, therefore, is not associated with the left hand side of the self-determined behaviour continuum. It is about ensuring continuous learning, persistence, interest, creativity, energy, well-being, sense of competence, autonomy and belonging that grow as you move towards the right hand end of the continuum. These are the things that will deliver sustained high performance.

Use Time-Out 6.2 below to reflect on your motivation at work and where it lies on the continuum shown in Figure 6.1. Think about the implications and impact it has on you and your performance.

Time-Out 6.2

To what extent do you determine your motivation and behaviour?

- Where are you on the purely external-purely internal continuum when you're at work?
- Does where you lie on the continuum vary across situation and demand?
- How does this influence your ability to deliver sustained high performance?
- How does it influence your ability to bounce back from performance setbacks?
- How much pressure and stress do you experience as a result of where your motivation lies?

It would be unrealistic and inappropriate in most performance contexts for you to be purely internally-motivated. The stakes are simply just too high in business for performers to be permitted to pursue and satisfy their personal needs solely for interest and enjoyment, but you can focus on achieving an optimal *degree* of self-determined behaviour. This is a function of how you are able to align the external motivators with your own values and motives, and also considering what you can do about the social environment in which you perform. Some of the strategies for achieving a greater sense of self-determination in the environment you currently operate in include the following:

- Ensuring that goals that are externally-imposed include short-term goals that allow you to monitor progress on a regular basis, thus gradually building your feeling of competence.
- Requesting regular feedback on your development that will similarly provide a means of monitoring your progress.
- Testing how much autonomy you have over your behaviour, and demonstrating that you want and are capable of more as appropriate.
- Getting to know your fellow performers as people and not just team members.
- Involving yourself, where you can, in decisions around future strategy.
- Involving yourself in the day-to-day operation of key factors in the performance environment.
- Taking time to fully understand the meaning and importance of tasks you are asked to carry out but do not enjoy.

All of the strategies above are aimed at satisfying your basic needs of competence, autonomy and relatedness. There will be other ways of developing greater self-determination of behaviour that will be specific to you and the environment you are performing in. Spend some time thinking about what these might be.

So what is optimal motivation?

To say that high performers are highly motivated is a statement of the obvious. However, extremely high levels of motivation may be necessary to repeatedly produce the kind of quality performance that will place you amongst the real elite. There is much to be learned from high level sport performers in this respect. Their ability to maintain motivation throughout the duration of a gruelling season, during periods of enforced rest through injury, and following setbacks in training and competition is a characteristic of the very best which distinguishes them from those who are merely 'very good'. But it is not just the *level* of motivation that is important; it is also the *nature* of motivation that is so influential. It should be clear from the previous sections that there are several factors to consider and regulate in order to optimise your motivation. Just to remind you, the key characteristics of optimal motivation are these.

- Approach rather than avoidance – ensure your motivation is about what you want to do rather than what you are trying to get away from.
- Active rather than passive – don't wait for things to happen, make them happen yourself.
- Do it for yourself rather than for others – satisfy your own needs before you can satisfy others as you would like.
- Positive rather than negative – ensure your motivation is about enjoyment rather than desperation.
- Internal rather than external – try to focus on the pride, enjoyment, interest and satisfaction you derive from achieving, as opposed to just the tangible rewards you receive for being successful.
- Self-determined – in situations and circumstances where you are driven by the external rewards for success, try to achieve as much autonomy over your behaviour as possible.

Don't worry if your motivation to perform doesn't fit all the characteristics above, because it is an ideal list. But recognise the nature of your motivation, where it may deviate from the optimal and reflect on it. Some subtle changes to how you think about achieving and being successful could have a big impact.

Over to Adrian . . .

I always remember when I was a child my parents being active in making things happen and this was a lesson that was part of the way we were bought up. My father was a good role model for me in overcoming potential hurdles that his background would have caused him. I can remember coming back from school once whinging about something (I can't recall exactly what it was) not going my way. One of my parents said 'don't wait for someone to do it for you, go and do it for yourself.' The other important thing in our family was the feeling that you shouldn't do something just to please other people. I never felt like I was doing something just to satisfy my parents; they were supportive whether I won or lost my races.

When I describe the training regime of a competitive swimmer to people (getting up at five o'clock in the morning, swimming for two hours before school and the two hours after school etc!), they often tell me that it must have been such a sacrifice, but I never looked at it like that. I always believed I was making a choice. For three years, before I got my driving licence, my father drove me to training at five o'clock in the morning, and never once if I slept through my alarm did he wake me up, i.e. he wasn't going to make me go, it was my choice. He just went back to bed!

→ Self-determining your motivation through setting goals

I have referred briefly to setting goals as being an important part of the process of developing mental toughness. This section takes a detailed look at goal setting because it is so inextricably linked to motivation.

We all set goals, but some people may not always be aware of it and so are often uncertain as to precisely what they are. This can mean that some performers become easily distracted and derailed under pressure as they lack a specific frame of reference to harness their focus. My experience of elite sport performers is that they set goals in a structured and meticulous fashion. Goals help these performers make sense of what they are trying to achieve and engender persistence in the most arduous circumstances. Goals provide the drive and discipline for performers to persevere in the face of adversity and to bounce back after failure. They provide a focus for performers who might otherwise become distracted when the pressure is really on. And they provide a huge sense of confidence when they are achieved.

What are the key essentials of setting effective goals? I have deliberately used the term 'effective goals' to emphasise that not all goals are effective and can actually be dysfunctional. There is a fine dividing line between setting goals that are just about achievable, but with a level of uncertainty that sustains your motivation, focus and effort, and those goals that are unattainable and actually add to the already intense pressure performers may find themselves under. Such goals are ultimately demotivating and counterproductive.

INSPIRED Goals

I refer to effective goals as 'inspired' goals since they satisfy a number of important criteria that can be identified under the acronym INSPIRED. The key elements of INSPIRED goals are that they should be:

- **I**nternalised
- **N**urturing
- **S**pecific
- **P**lanned
- **I**n your control
- **R**eviewed regularly
- **E**nergising
- **D**ocumented

Some pointers for developing INSPIRED goals are as follows:

Internalised

No matter who has set your goals for you, it is important that you own and commit to them if they are to be effective. If your goals have been set by others, then you should internalise and integrate them so that they become meaningful and worthwhile, thus resulting in a greater sense of self-determination over your behaviour. When goals are accepted and internalised, performance generally increases as goals become more difficult. Conversely, when goals are rejected performance drops off as they become more difficult.

Nurturing

Effective goals are those where the process is not merely about delivering against targets; they also provide an opportunity for learning and further development. This means that goals should include a developmental element so that significant learning occurs in addition to targets being achieved. This helps you satisfy current goals as well as ensuring continual progress towards even higher levels of performance.

Specific

Effective goals are clear and unambiguous so that it is obvious when they have been achieved. This does not necessarily mean that they have to be quantifiable. Effective goals can be set around things like confidence or focus, areas that are very difficult to attach numbers to. But such goals can be specific in the sense that certain thoughts and actions can be aimed for.

Planned

There are two aspects of breaking down and planning goals that are important; time frame, and ensuring that different types of goals are aligned with more overriding goals that drive your motivation. I will deal with aligning different goal types in the following section because this lies at the very core of motivation and delivering sustained high performance. In the context of time frame, short-term goals plus long-term goals leads to higher performance than long-term goals alone. The importance of building short-term or sub-goals into the 'goal achievement plan' is that they provide immediate incentives and feedback and the attainment of sub-goals provides evidence of competence, thus resulting in enhanced confidence.

In your control

For goals to be highly motivating on a sustainable basis, the achievement of them should be attainable through your own efforts. This does not mean that you should not have goals that focus on coming out ahead of your comepetitors, whose performance you cannot control; indeed, these are the very things that underpin many goal setting strategies. Being in control refers, instead, to the fact that effective goals should not be at the mercy of extraneous factors such as market forces or the weather that really are uncontrollable.

Reviewed regularly

Effective goals form part of the longer-term continued development and growth of high achievers. Because of the sometimes prolonged nature of this process, regular reviews of progress towards longer-term goals should be included in the planning process. Also, key sources and methods of obtaining feedback should be identified and built into the goal setting plan.

Energising

Goals should excite and energise you, and they should produce a great sense of achievement when they are attained. For goals to satisfy these criteria, they must be challenging in that they are just about achievable, but with a level of uncertainty that sustains your motivation, focus and effort.

Documented

Having got all the other elements of effective goal setting right, it would be a shame if it all fell down because this final element was ignored. Documenting the goals in some form and recording progress towards them provides a continual reminder of commitments that can be important when things are tough. It helps you to step outside any pressure and remind yourself why you are doing it and why it is all worthwhile. Ideally, your goals should be constantly visible, perhaps carried around in your organiser or wallet. Some sport performers I have worked with have put them on their bedroom wall, ensuring that they wake each morning with a meaningful focus for the day.

Ensuring different goal types are aligned: outcome, performance and process goals

A key factor in planning goals is to ensure that different types of goal are aligned towards the same ends. There are three different types of goals that form the basis of motivation: outcome, performance and process goals.

- **Outcome goals** focus on the outcomes of particular events and usually involve interpersonal comparison of some kind; for example, winning a 400 metre hurdles race.
- **Performance goals** specify an end product of performance that will be achieved by the performer independently of other performers; for example, running the 400 metre hurdle race in a certain time.
- **Process goals** focus on processes that are important during the performance; for example, maintaining a good lead leg technique over each hurdle.

Adrian explains below how breaking his performance down in this way was a crucial part of his success.

Over to Adrian . . .

Breaking my performance down into these three components enabled me to win my Gold Medal in the 1988 Seoul Olympics. My performance would first of all clearly be measured against whether I achieved my desired outcome – the Gold Medal. This provided me with a specific time frame and a dream that formed the core of my passion, inspiration and the desire that drove me, particularly when things were not going my way. This outcome goal involved an interpersonal, competitive element in that I had to beat seven opponents in the Olympic final to win the Gold Medal.

I was not completely in control of this goal, of course, since I could have swum brilliantly but still have been beaten by other swimmers who had swum even more brilliantly. Therefore, I set a performance goal that I could totally control. I reckoned that a time of 62 seconds or better would be good enough to win the Gold Medal. All of my training and practice was geared towards swimming this time. My performance goals during the four years prior to the Olympics were mapped out in terms of the various times, or milestones, that were required at various points along the journey. These goals provided me with a sense of achievement, self-belief and sustained motivation as I monitored my progress towards the ultimate performance goal of 62 seconds.

In order to achieve this performance I focused on specific underlying process goals, such as improving my turning technique at the end of each length and my reaction to the starting gun. Process goals like these formed the very foundation of achieving my performance goal of 62 seconds. The numerous processes practised over and over again on a daily basis in training drove my continual dedication, commitment, focus and sheer effort at times when you were probably tucked up in your warm, comfortable beds. The process goals were subject to continual monitoring and review, with detailed contingency plans that could be implemented when progress strayed off course.

One process I particularly focused on was 'holding my technique' during the last ten metres of a race. The 100 metre breaststroke is essentially a sprint event in which swimmers become fatigued and lose their technique as the race nears its end. I focused on keeping my stroke technique smooth during those last few metres. As events transpired, coming into the last few metres of the race in fourth place, I finished with technique intact and passed my three opponents to win by a fingernail.

What Adrian had done was to plan his success by aligning outcome, performance and process goals in the fashion shown in Figure 6.2. Goals planned in this meticulous and aligned fashion provide performers with a crucial tool for maintaining psychological control when the pressure of competing is at its most ferocious. They also serve as a much needed reference that helps performers cope with the daily grind and monotony of training. There are numerous other similar stories of how sport performers have achieved great things by breaking performance down into outcome, performance and process goals, and the principles apply equally well in the business environment.

A sales executive I worked with defined a successful outcome goal as winning the prestigious Salesperson of the Year award. She was obviously in competition with her 120 colleagues and thus not in control of this outcome, no matter how good her sales figures were for the year. What she *was* in control over was her level of personal performance and, following careful consideration, she concentrated her efforts on achieving figures that bettered her previous year's numbers by 15 per cent. She identified some key processes underpinning this improvement, the most important of which was to modify her philosophy on the selling process. She wanted to become someone who a customer 'bought from' rather than was 'sold to'. This determined her approach to the customer experience and she achieved a 17 per cent improvement on the previous year's figures. She came second to a colleague who had had an even more impressive year, but she felt good about what she had achieved and how she had done it, and entered the following year both confident and motivated.

Figure 6.2 Aligning outcome, performance and process goals.

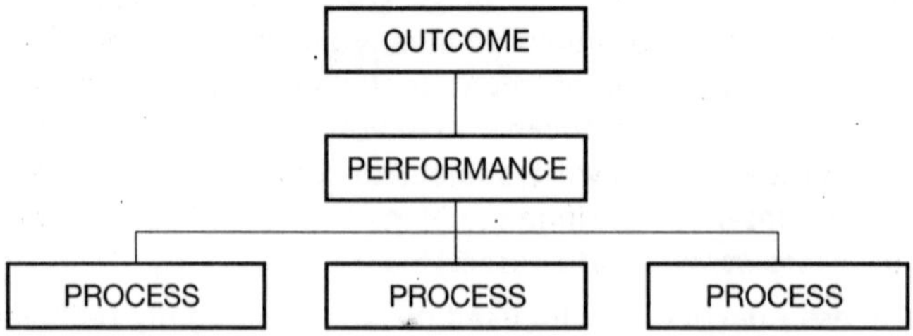

Knowing how to plan different types of goals that are aligned to outcomes is therefore key to achieving high performance that is sustainable. Figure 6.3 provides a detailed example of how linking process, performance and outcome goals enabled a manager to plan his career development. The outcome goal he identified was to achieve a senior leadership role within three years. He then identified performance goals in eight areas (being visionary, an influencer, decisive, a team builder, credible, having presence, being confident and achieving a good work-life balance) that would ensure his progress towards the outcome goal, and also that he could totally control. The next stage was to identify process goals that underpinned the delivery of each performance goal. These process goals provided his day-to-day focus, and we built in a measurement and regular review process that enabled him to monitor his progress towards his performance goals.

Figure 6.3 **Aligning outcome, performance and process goals: an example.**

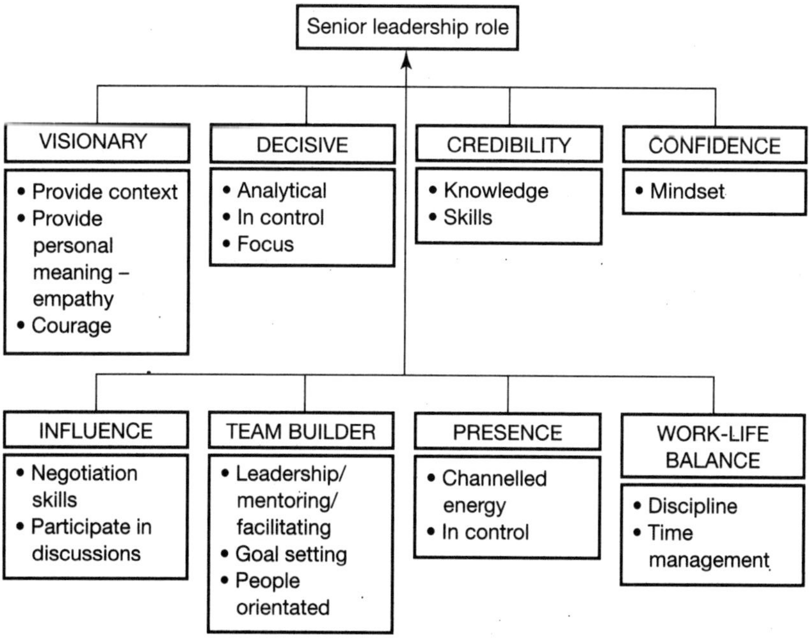

The important things to remember are that performance should be planned in a top-down fashion, identifying the desired outcome, associated performances and the key underlying processes that will enable them to be achieved. When it comes to carrying out the plan on a day-to-day basis, then a bottom-up approach is required, focusing on processes first. It is the continual focus on getting the processes right that will eventually deliver the performances and outcomes.

Over to Adrian . . .

The use of different goal types has been one of the biggest revelations of my life! It is one of the most useful pieces of knowledge that I have ever been aware of and I use it to this day. The use of outcome, performance and process goals gives a structure to achieving performance, whether it be winning swimming races, learning a new language or winning a business deal. The idea is that it's ok to set an outcome goal, something you really want, that will motivate you if you get it. But then it's vital that you break it down into measurable performance and most importantly the processes that you will use to get there; eventually these processes become part of your daily routine.

I have already described how I used this in swimming, but right now this goal structure drives our business' strategy. We have a series of outcome statements for the business, and all the performance goals that most companies have around revenues, profitability, etc. But it's the process goals that sit with the different departments and individuals in the business and this is where we take control of our performance and have more chance of achieving.

For me, the crucial aspect of this tool is not just the hard framework, but the emotional link to motivation. It gives you the opportunity to stretch yourself and others in a variety of different areas that can play to the motivations of the individual. Also, when we review progress, we don't have just one numerical goal that can be a success or failure. We have more richness in the type of achievements we might have made, particularly in the process area.

Now that you know about INSPIRED goals and the importance of achieving outcome goals via aligned performance and process goals, apply these frameworks in Time-Out 6.3 below to help you plan the achievement of your own career aspirations.

Time-Out 6.3

Planning your future

1. What do you want to achieve in the future, and when? (e.g. senior leadership role in the next three years).
2. What are the performance goals that will ensure progress towards your outcome goal? Make sure that they are things that you can totally control (e.g. being visionary, an influencer, decisive, a team builder, credible, having presence, being confident and achieving a good work-life balance).

3. What are the process goals that will underpin the delivery of each performance goal? These process goals should provide a day-to-day focus (e.g. being a team builder might be underpinned by coaching and mentoring, setting goals and being people-orientated).
4. How will you measure and review your progress?

Ensure that your goals are INSPIRED goals – **I**(nternalised), **N**(urturing), **S**(pecific), **P**(lanned), **I**(n your control), **R**(eviewed regularly), **E**(nergising), **D**(ocumented).

Chris Andy Scott Emma Studies

Chris

Chris had reached a point where he was seriously considering handing in his resignation following another painful defeat. Nothing he tried was making a difference; he felt helpless and had lost his strong sense of competence and autonomy. Chris had become acquiescent to media calls for a different game strategy and player selections. He also felt worn down by a constant political power struggle amongst influential stakeholders that made his job even harder. Both he and the team now seemed devoid of purpose and direction.

Chris was horrified at his subsequent realisation that he was showing some classic signs of the beginnings of learned helplessness. He began the task of clawing back greater self-determination by setting short-term goals around dealing with the constraints he had identified in the demands/supports/constraints exercise described in Chapter 4. He also focused on maximising his supports and set goals around those too. In the context of the team, Chris worked with them on establishing an outcome goal in the form of a vision for the next three years. This was accompanied by setting initial performance goals around games scheduled over the next few months. Finally, a series of process goals was established and agreed around the attitudes and behaviours of all concerned, including the support staff. This provided a clear sense of purpose as well as a day-to-day focus that became valuable for restoring a sense of self-determined motivation and behaviour.

Andy

Andy's motivation was underpinned by the pressure and ensuing stress resulting from the huge expectations on him, as well as his perception that his colleagues did not respect or value his leadership capability. He was not enjoying the situation at all and he reached a point where most of his time was devoted to avoiding failure; and his performance suffered because he had become fearful of assuming the leadership role the business required. His colleagues had become enemies in his eyes, and he was suspicious of their every action.

Andy worked on dealing with his avoidance motivation by first of all recognising the need to assume some level of self-determination rather than merely letting the situation and circumstances continue. He identified short-term process goals that would improve working relationships and restore a sense of relatedness and belonging to his direct report team. These goals focused around literally 'approaching' his colleagues so that he could get to know them at a personal level, as well as learning to value their comments and opinions in personal interactions. Andy's goals also focused on 'how to be' as a leader, in terms of his presence, his chairing of meetings, etc. These goals gave a meaning to his behaviour that he was able to internalise and gain a much stronger sense of self-determination.

Scott

Scott's motivation was founded on his desperation to obtain sufficient money to pay off his debts and earn a decent living. Only one thing, in his eyes, would satisfy this need - winning the next and every tournament he entered. His motivation had become purely external; he needed to win at any cost, and with it came intense stress. He clearly needed to regain some self-determination over his motivation and behaviour. Through what was quite a tough process of rationalising the situation he was in, Scott acknowledged that his goal of winning every tournament he entered was unrealistic and not within his control. What *was* within his control was his own performance and the processes underpinning it. An important part of the goal setting process involved reminding himself that being a professional golfer was something he once dreamed about and that golf was once a huge source of enjoyment for him.

Scott worked through setting goals based on outcomes, performances and processes. His outcome goal for the season was quite simply to keep his card so that he could play on the professional tour the following year. Performance goals were set around things within his control, such as average number of putts and number of fairways hit per round. Process goals focused on things like establishing a consistent pre-shot routine that would be robust under the most severe pressure, as well as remaining composed and confident. Thinking about his process and performance goals actually helped to alleviate the stress he was under because he was able to see how he could control his thoughts and behaviours through a sense of self-determination, rather than being controlled by the environment and circumstances he found himself in.

Emma

Emma's motives to succeed were founded on a self-imposed pressure that she had to prove herself within a male-dominated environment. In essence, she had little self-determination over her behaviour; she was behaving in a manner that she thought she ought to, and not necessarily how she wanted to. Her motivation was towards the external end of the motivation continuum and she needed to instil some internal motivation in the form of greater self-determination.

Emma needed to focus on things like her own pride, satisfaction and enjoyment as the motives to be a good performer and leader. She needed to do it for herself, not to prove herself to others. She found hearing about and reading some of the research literature on high-achieving female leaders really helpful in understanding the important attributes that females bring to the leader role. This all pointed towards the importance of being herself and not someone or something else that she thought was expected of her. Her subsequent new focus on the process of enjoying the role and personal growth reduced much of the stress she had been under and she became a much more 'natural' leader with a far greater sense of self-determination.

In a nutshell

- The very best performers are not driven by fear of failure (i.e. avoidance motivation); instead, they are driven by the desire for success (i.e. approach motivation).
- For performers who are externally-motivated over prolonged periods, their internal motivation subsides so that they become heavily dependent on material rewards to keep going.
- The further you are towards the external end of the external-internal motivation continuum, the more pressure and potential stress there is to perform to others' high expectations.
- Mental toughness is about ensuring that you do not stray too far from the internal, complete self-determination end of the motivation continuum.
- Optimal motivation constitutes approach, active, self-focused, positive, internal and self-regulated motives.
- Identifying 'effective', INSPIRED goals is an important part of the process of developing mental toughness.

What next?

- Develop strategies for achieving a greater sense of self-determination in the environment you currently operate in.
- Find ways of feeling competent in what you do, exercising choice over your behaviour, and relating in some positive way to the people you are performing with and/or the cause you are contributing to.
- Set effective goals that will deliver sustained high motivation and performance via **I**(nternalised), **N**(urturing), **S**(pecific), **P**(lanned), **I**(n your control), **R**(eviewed regularly), **E**(nergising), **D**(ocumented) goals.
- Plan your performances by setting aligned outcome, performance and process goals.

7 Maintaining Your Focus on the Things that Matter

After reading this chapter you will know about:

- What you *should* be focused on
- How to shut out distractions
- How to switch your focus

I remember reading about baseball legend Babe Ruth when he was in a batting slump and his team was in danger of being knocked out of the World Series. He was two strikes down and received some abuse from a particularly loud spectator behind the batting plate. His response was to hit a home run off the next pitch. He was later asked what he was thinking about as he stood on the plate with only one chance left. Was he thinking about the guy in the crowd who was giving him a hard time? Was he thinking about the pressure on him because he would be out if he missed the next pitch? Was he thinking about the crisis his team was in? Ruth told them that none of these things entered his head and that he was simply thinking about one thing only – hitting the ball!

Focus is a relatively straightforward requirement of high performance made complex by the fact that there are just so many things you could focus on. For Babe Ruth, there were a number of things he could have been focusing on as the pitcher was winding up to release the ball, and he could have fallen into the trap of focusing on things that were merely distractions. The simple focus required was on the ball and hitting it. People often over-complicate things by focusing on extraneous factors that threaten to intrude on their performance. This chapter shows you how to recognise what you should focus on and how to maintain your focus on the things that matter.

Over to Adrian . . .

Focus is one of the key areas that requires practice even at the very highest levels. When you are about to dive in for a world championship final, you must be totally focused on the job in hand. I suppose that I must have learned through the years how to manage all the distractions, so much so that it is now a subconscious thing. I think that I box things in my head. I now categorise them as useful or not useful to me in the moment. I make split second decisions, and if the information, or noise, or email is not relevant in that moment then I put it away until I can deal with it. It is the art of staying in the moment, and the key is realising that you have total control of how you interpret external information.

→ Are you focused on your focus?

Take a few moments to think about what happens to your focus when you are under pressure.

- Are you so completely focused on your performance that nothing else matters?
- Or are you easily distracted?
- Now think about what you would like to achieve by reading this chapter.
- By the way, what are you doing tomorrow?
- And what else is going on in your life right now?

Have I distracted you from the purpose of reading this chapter? If you have carefully followed the instructions and questions above, then I have shifted your focus around so it has not necessarily been where you wanted or planned. So you may have been focused, but perhaps not always on the things that will help you achieve your aim! That's what happens to your focus. There are so many different things fighting for its attention that it's sometimes very difficult to keep it directed towards those things that matter. And it's even harder to remain focused on the things that really matter when the pressure is on. Pressure, in itself, can be a major threat to your focus. Thinking about the consequences of failure or how you *must* be successful, for example, distracts you from focusing on the very things that really matter in delivering the performance you are aiming for.

Distractions are sometimes caused by things that have happened in the past that you just cannot let go of. Elwyn was a long-serving senior manager and high performer in a business that was undergoing a structural re-organisation which would mean having to deliver even higher performance with fewer resources. The change involved introducing a new matrix management structure which resulted in one of Elwyn's former peers being promoted to a position into which he now reported. Elwyn liked his new manager at a personal level and had always got on well with him as a peer, but two things bothered him about the new situation: firstly, he felt the new management position was unnecessary and created further bureaucracy in the form of yet another layer of decision-making; and secondly, he believed he was more capable than his new manager and was both confused and angry about being overlooked for the position.

Our coaching sessions became dominated by Elwyn's failure to accept the situation. It was clear that his focus was not on his day-to-day performance, but on the circumstances surrounding the earlier re-structure. Here was a classic case of someone who was focusing on the wrong things and, worse still, it was having a debilitating effect on his performance.

The same can happen in sport where performers sometimes focus on things that will *not* help and often impair their performance. Rugby players who focus on *not* dropping the first pass they receive, or golfers who focus on *not* hitting the ball into the bunker to the right of the green often end up doing those very things. And the rugby player who *does* drop a try-scoring pass in the first few minutes of a big game might spend the rest of it focusing on this 'catastrophic' mistake. Likewise, the golfer in the bunker might be focusing on frustration and anger at being in it rather than on the vital recovery shot. If focusing on the mistakes they have just made is not enough to distract these performers, then focusing on the future is another danger to delivering optimum performance. The rugby player may spend the remainder of the game worrying about what tomorrow's newspapers will make of his vital error. The golfer in the bunker may be focusing on how crucial the next shot is in securing a much-needed big pay cheque.

The examples of Elwyn, the rugby player and the golfer demonstrate how it is very easy to be distracted from delivering your best performance. They also illustrate how it is not just events and factors in the current environment that are competing for your attention; past and future events, and how you think about them, can also dominate your focus and impair your performance – if you let them!

So what should you be focused on?

'Focus' is one of those words used frequently and freely to embrace a multitude of things involved in delivering high level performance. A bit like the term 'mental toughness' really; most people have a vague sense of what it is, but few are able to clearly define it. In its simplest form, 'focus' is about clear and vivid thoughts and images that occupy your conscious mind, and involves withdrawing thoughts and images from some things to deal effectively with others.

A recurring theme throughout this book has been self-awareness, and so it continues in the context of enhancing your ability to achieve 'appropriate focus'. Appropriate focus involves directing your thinking towards what you *should* be thinking about. This all sounds very obvious and merely common sense. But common sense is not always common practice, particularly in the case of focus. I'm sure you know that it is not a particularly good idea to think about the mistakes you might make during the final minutes and moments before an important presentation, negotiation or interview. Instead, you *should* be focusing on things like how well prepared you are, the opportunity (as opposed to threat) that lies ahead, the skills and abilities that you have at your disposal, and so on. But people like myself are in demand because some performers struggle to understand what to focus on and/or how to control their focus.

The content of the focus you are trying to achieve is a function of numerous factors, which means that an 'appropriate focus' can vary enormously from situation to situation, from individual to individual and from second to second. It is difficult to generalise, therefore, but high achievers from a wide variety of sports consistently report the following as being important.

- **Controlling the controllables** – this is an often-used phrase and emphasises the futility of devoting any of that valuable, limited-capacity focus to things that you just cannot control. Mentally tough performers accept that there are factors in the performance environment they cannot influence, identify what they are and then focus on the things they can control.
- **Focusing on process** – high level performance is about getting the processes right. The key processes underpinning performance have already been identified earlier in this book as something that mentally tough performers use as an important source of internal motivation to

drive them to practise and prepare thoroughly and meticulously. They also provide a fundamental focus during performance itself – focus on the processes of performing and the outcomes will take care of themselves.

- **Staying in the moment** – during performance, it is very important (in most circumstances) to focus on what is happening in the moment. I have already described earlier in the chapter how it makes no sense to focus on mistakes; they are history. You can do nothing to change them so why beat yourself up about them? Accept they have happened, 'bin' them and move on. Similarly, looking into the future can be a distraction. Some golfers who find themselves five-under-par after seven holes can get carried away by thoughts of a very low score. That's almost as bad as being five-over and thinking they're going to score in the 80s, rather than focusing on what they have to do right here and how.
- **Focusing on positives** – if external distractions are not enough to disrupt your focus, then internal ones lurk menacingly in the background. Thoughts of past failures in similar circumstances to those you find yourself in, the consequences of failure or your doubts about being able to achieve your performance goals are all examples of negative thoughts that are unhelpful. Focusing on things such as your past achievements and things you're particularly good at is much more conducive to a positive state of readiness to perform well.
- **Fire in the belly, ice in the head** – because of the pressure associated with delivering high performance when it really matters, simply focusing on remaining composed when the adrenaline is pumping can be a very effective strategy. I described in Chapter 4 how a quick relaxation technique based on focusing on a mantra or keyword, such as 'relax' or 'calm', as you breathe out is very helpful in achieving a composed state. Think about using that technique as a way to help you control your focus when under pressure.

You will need to apply and adapt these key pointers to achieving an appropriate focus to the specific set of conditions and circumstances that exist in your own performance environment. They will serve as useful prompts and reminders of the things you *should* be focusing on when the pressure is on.

Over to Adrian . . .

One of the key messages in this section is the aspect of 'control'. All five of the above points have control at the heart of them. The one example I have that sums this up is that moment *immediately* before the race is about to begin, and I mean the last 30 seconds before the gun goes off. At that point I can only control the next thing that is about to happen to me, and that is the dive into the pool. I have no impact on my rivals. I cannot change my previous races. I can only impact on the way I enter the pool. I get on to the block visualising the best dive I have ever done. I wait, and as the gun goes off, I am thinking about squeezing the block, tipping my body weight forward and launching at about 45 degrees, driving through my legs with all the force I can. Then I do the next thing . . . I've started.

Focus and mental toughness

The problem with focus is that there is simply not enough of it to enable you to deal with all of the things demanding its attention. The conscious mind has a limited capacity and is only able to hold a relatively small amount of information at any one time. Read the following string of numbers *quickly* and once only, and then look away and write them down on a sheet of paper in the same order that they appear below.

7	2	0	9	6	3	1	4	8	5

How many did you get right? The likelihood is that you got at least one wrong because remembering a string of ten numbers in the correct sequence will overload the conscious minds of the vast majority of people. Even if you did write the numbers down in the correct order, you would not have been able to think about anything else whilst you were recalling them. Given that the capacity of the conscious mind is so limited, then what you put or allow into it is pretty important.

Being able to control the content of the conscious mind so that it is able to achieve optimum focus involves getting rid of inappropriate thoughts and replacing them with appropriate ones, as shown in Figure 7.1. For example, negative thoughts in the form of worry and self-doubt are unlikely to be helpful to performers who, instead, want to think positively and confidently about their upcoming performance. The inappropriate, negative thoughts that are doing their best to impair your performance therefore need to be banished and replaced by more appropriate, positive thoughts that will help you perform well.

Figure 7.1 Gaining control over your thoughts.

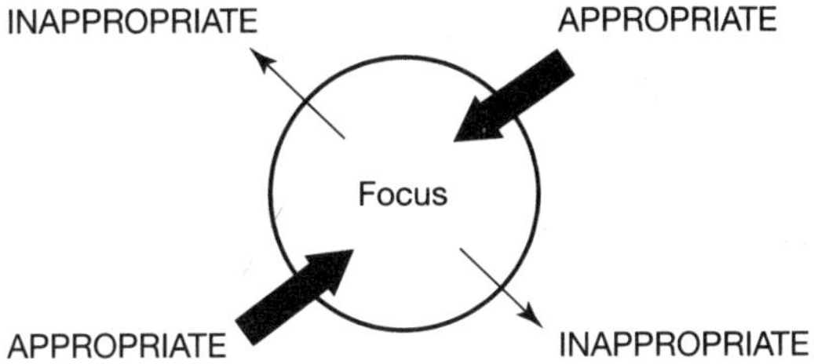

Focus, therefore, is a limited capacity resource that you must use and implement very carefully indeed if you are to optimise your performance. Performers who are mentally tough have high levels of control over their focus and where they direct it. Our research with high achievers in both sport and business shows that mental toughness involves being able to maintain, and sometimes regain, an appropriate focus at times when it is being seriously threatened. These research findings indicate a number of aspects of focus that are key to being mentally tough:

- being able to shut out the 'usual' distractions that you expect in your performance environment;
- being able to recover from unexpected, uncontrollable events;
- ensuring that you are not distracted by others' performance and focus only on your own performance;
- being able to focus on your performance when there are other things going on in your life;
- re-energising your performance focus when required;
- not getting derailed by success and failure.

These aspects of focus, together with related strategies and techniques for maintaining and regaining focus, are described below.

Shutting out the 'usual' distractions in your performance environment

There are a multitude of 'things' in the performance environment competing for your attention that will impair your performance if you fall into the trap of directing some or all of your limited focus towards them. For the most part, these distractions are usually predictable in that they 'go with the territory'. Typical examples in sport include crowd noise, poor refereeing decisions and an opponent who might be trying to psyche you out. The equivalent at work will be specific to your situation and circumstances, but may typically include things like continual interruptions by colleagues and receiving a mountain of emails that all seem to require urgent responses.

So how can you ensure that your focus is on those things that really matter? The important thing about dealing with these types of distractions is not to be surprised and to plan how to manage them. Here are three simple strategies and techniques that you can employ.

1 **Accept the existence of distractions**. Accept potential distractions as a natural part of the performance environment; they exist and there is often little you can do about them. Don't *try* to ignore them – this effort alone will take up some of that valuable focus. Instead, let thoughts of them pass and return to what you want to focus on. You will grow accustomed to encountering distractions and therefore not be surprised by them.

2 **Recognise distractions – identify what matters**. The key to not being distracted from your performance is to recognise distractions and when you are focusing on them. For Elwyn, the senior manager introduced earlier in this chapter, focusing on his frustration and confusion about being overlooked for a more senior role was both wasteful and futile. It was wasteful in the sense that he was directing his limited capacity focus away from things that would help his performance to something that was causing him stress and distracting him from performing optimally. Furthermore, it was futile because there was nothing Elwyn could do to reverse the situation – it was history and out of his control. What he should have been focused on were the things under his control that would ensure sustainable, high level performance.

3 **'Am I focusing on what really matters?'** This simple question acts as a trigger to re-focusing, if necessary, on the things that matter. Some executives I work with have learned to associate seeing small self-adhesive coloured dots with asking themselves the question 'am I

focusing on what really matters?', and have stuck them on frequently used things such as phones or computer screens. This was a really useful technique for Elwyn whose carefully placed dots became a trigger for him to recognise when his frustration was getting in the way, and to then re-focus on the things that mattered to delivering the performance he aimed for. Sports performers who have experienced similar difficulties in 'tuning in' to the right things have also benefited from this technique.

Over to Adrian . . .

As I have already mentioned, one of my techniques for staying focused was to put away external distractions if they were not useful to the current job in hand. However, one of the hardest things to block out was the crowd noise. In the end, I decided that my usual technique just wasn't going to work. It's hard to block out 18,000 screaming people! My revised strategy was to acknowledge it was there, and I did two things: firstly, I imagined that they were all screaming for me (despite the different national flags!); and secondly, I 'turned it down' to become nice background 'music'.

Use Time-Out 7.1 below to jot down those things that are common distractions in your own performance environment and then reflect on how you might deal with them more effectively.

Time-Out 7.1

Shutting out the 'usual' distractions in your performance environment

- What are the 'usual' distractions that exist in your performance environment?
- What are the things that really matter to your performance and that you can control?
- Think of a trigger that will stimulate you to ask the question 'am I focusing on what really matters?'

Recovering from unexpected, uncontrollable events

Sometimes, distractions can be unexpected and uncontrollable; they appear from nowhere and can completely derail you. And it does not have to be a negative event that threatens your focus. A hole-in-one in golf is a classic example of having to regain focus after an unexpected case of exceptionally good performance. Potential derailers I have come across in the business world include events such as the unexpected announcement of the sale of the company, or discovering that your slide presentation has been wiped from your laptop computer minutes before a pitch for a substantial piece of business. Worse still can be the discovery that a direct report has just made a mistake that will cost the company a lot of money.

The key in these circumstances is to regain your composure as quickly as possible and to continue with minimal disruption towards your desired goal. Business executives can learn a lot from elite sport performers who have developed a number of techniques and strategies for such situations. Three of the more effective ones are described below.

What ifs. This technique involves identifying mainly those things that could go wrong, and occasionally those that could be distracting because things go much better than anticipated, such as the hole-in-one in golf. Extending the golf analogy a little further, the goal of golfers on any hole other than a par three is almost exclusively to strike the ball so that it comes to rest on the fairway. The best golfers I have worked with rehearse 'what ifs' such as 'what if I hit it in the thick rough on the right on this hole?' or 'what if my ball ends up in the deep bunker 180 yards short of the green?' They work out what they would do in these tricky circumstances before they encounter them; they have plans that effectively take the decision-making out of the heat of the situation when the pressure may cause them to take a rash course of action.

Simulations. A world-ranked racket sport player I worked with was well known for losing her focus when the pressure was on and things started to go wrong. Whether it was what she thought was a bad call by the umpire, or a particularly bad shot she had just played, she was unable to put thoughts of what had just happened out of her mind. We set up situations where she would play practice games against training partners in which an umpire was primed to give bad calls against her. Whilst this did not simulate competitive playing conditions exactly, it was effective in providing a safe environment in which she could learn and practise a different and more constructive way of responding to such situations in the future.

Mental rehearsal. As well as setting up physical simulations of specific circumstances within the competitive environment, the racket sport player also used mental rehearsal to help her learn to re-focus when things went wrong. She imagined herself playing a bad shot and then being able to shut thoughts of the shot out of her mind, before re-focusing on the next rally. This technique proved effective and convenient because she could practise it frequently and in many different types of circumstances.

The techniques described above may seem and sound a little strange in the world of business where such things may seem a bit 'touchy-feely'. I can only encourage you to experiment with them; you may be surprised at how effective they can be in helping you remain composed and focused even in the most trying of circumstances. Use Time-Out 7.2 below to jot down some ideas about how you might employ them.

Time-Out 7.2

Recovering from unexpected, uncontrollable events

- What ifs - what are the things that could go wrong, or even extremely well, that you would not expect and would be uncontrollable in your quest to deliver high performance on a sustainable basis? What would you do if any of these potential events occurred?
- Simulations - are there any ways you can simulate the 'what ifs' so that you can enact how you would respond?
- Mental rehearsal - go through your planned response in your mind until you are confident that it is sufficiently ingrained that you would *actually* respond in that way. Do this on a regular basis.

Over to Adrian . . .

In sport I always used to mentally rehearse. It was useful in the Olympic final in 1988 when I turned in sixth out of eight with one length to go. I had actually prepared for that eventuality and knew exactly what my strategy was (specific stroke technique). Now in business, I find myself thinking about the eventualities, the 'what if' scenarios before any key business decision, or important sales meeting (call it 'daydreaming' if you like!). For instance, what are the hard questions that could be asked, what would my response be and how would I deliver it? To a large degree, all business strategy should have elements of scenario-planning.

Focusing on *your* performance only

Think about times when teammates or colleagues around you are struggling to deliver the performances they are capable of due to adverse conditions in the performance environment, perhaps in the form of a flat market or lack of resources. Does that mean that *you* perform at less than optimal levels as well? Mentally tough performers focus on performing at their best irrespective of how poorly others are performing, and without relying on a fallback position of being able to blame the conditions. This self-focus is not, though, a case of merely 'ploughing your own furrow' and being oblivious to what is going on around you. Mental toughness in this respect is about also spotting and providing support to those who are in need of it.

The key to focusing on *your* performance only lies in setting the different types of goals described in Chapter 6. To briefly recap, goals can be divided into outcome, performance and process goals. Outcome goals are essentially around winning or achieving some performance standard that is benchmarked against others' performance. Difficulties arise when outcome goals are the *only* ones that have been identified, with others' performance then having a big influence on your level of success. Being able to focus on *your* performance only involves identifying 'what' level of performance you want to achieve (i.e. performance goals) and 'how' to achieve it (i.e. process goals).

- **Focusing on 'what' you want to achieve.** Performance goals provide an important focus because they specify an end product that can be achieved independently of other performers – you're not in control over whether you win the race, but you *are* in control over how fast you run it! For elite sport performers, the performance is sometimes more important than the outcome; it is part of their development in their preparation for bigger events to come. Others' performances are not important in the grand scheme of things and they do not concern themselves with it.

- **Focusing on 'how' to achieve it**. Process goals involve focusing on the component parts of the performance. And they do not necessarily have to be about the physical or functional components – a focus on 'how to be' during a performance, such as 'confident' or 'relaxed' can be just as powerful. Whatever process(es) you focus on, this strategy ensures that your focus is not on others' performance and, instead, on things you can control.

Over to Adrian . . .

As I described in the last chapter, setting aligned outcome, performance and process goals was an important part of my Olympic success. The performance and process goals were particularly important because they helped me to focus on myself and not on the opposition. This was really important at times in competition when the pressure was intense.

Both of these strategies provide a focus that is about *you* and the things that *you* can control. They will enable you to maintain high levels of performance irrespective of how others are performing around you. Now spend a few minutes working through Time-Out 7.3.

Time-Out 7.3

Focusing on *your* performance only

- What are the things you want to achieve in your role on a day-to-day basis? These goals should be specific to the expectations of your role and independent of other people's performance.
- What are the processes that underpin the achievement of the goals identified above?
- How can you ensure that these goals will form your day-to-day focus irrespective of what is going on around you?

Focusing on performance when there are other things going on in your life

Mental toughness involves preventing events and circumstances in your personal life, both good and bad, from distracting you when performing. Relationships, births, deaths, financial affairs and the like are all important elements of life you cannot ignore, but there are times to focus on them and times to switch off from them! Being able to compartmentalise your life so that you can keep the various elements separate is an important aspect of being able to deliver sustainable high performance. Three techniques and strategies will help you in developing the ability to achieve this.

- **Setting time aside to deal with personal life distractions.** If you don't devote the necessary time to deal with issues outside the performance environment they will linger and be a constant source of potential distraction. Mental toughness involves setting quality time aside to tackle the issues head on rather than dealing with symptoms that never dissipate. Elite sports performers plan their time meticulously to fit in such non-performance-related activities.
- **Parking worries and coming back to them.** There will be times when you have to focus exclusively on your performance, but have those niggling thoughts in the background about personal life issues. Don't ignore them, because they won't go away. There are two slightly varying ways of dealing with them:

  1 Write your thoughts down on a piece of paper and put it in a secure place so you can come back to it at a time designated by yourself.

  2 Imagine yourself writing your thoughts down on a piece of paper and placing it in an imaginary box to deal with at a later time.

  Both methods provide the assurance that you will come back to them at a time that better suits you so you can put them out of your mind for the time being. The key is to 'park' any worries so they are not taken into the performance environment, but instead are dealt with at a more appropriate time.
- **Pressing the focus switch.** This is a simple technique which involves imagining a light switch which actually turns your performance focus on. All you do is imagine turning on the switch to focus you on the things that matter. A couple of performers I have worked with have actually carried a small light switch around with them to help them quite literally switch their performance focus on when required.

Over to Adrian . . .

One of the hardest things I had to deal with in this regard was coping with the death of one of my closest rivals, Victor Davis of Canada. He had already retired from swimming after the 1988 Olympics, with a career that included numerous Olympic and World Championship medals. A week before the Commonwealth Games selection trials in England, I heard that he had been killed in a car accident. It was made clear to me that I had to swim the trials in order to qualify for the team (at the time I was the World Record holder, but selection is never guaranteed). I found it really hard to deal with and was struggling to motivate myself to prepare in that last week.

Much as I knew how to, I couldn't box it away. I struggled to make the final – eighth qualifier, and in danger of missing the team. Just before the final, I sat down and remember thinking 'the race is only 60 seconds. You only have to block it out for a minute, then deal with it.' Somehow this worked, and I won the final and made the team.

These are simple techniques, but require some discipline in applying them. The key is to ensure you park thoughts about what is happening outside your performance arena and *always* return to deal with them; otherwise, these techniques will merely become convenient avoidance strategies that mean issues are never addressed head on. Have a go at figuring out how you can best deal with personal life distractions in Time-Out 7.4.

Time-Out 7.4

Focusing on performance when there are other things going on in your life

- Mental toughness involves setting quality time aside to tackle issues head on. What is going on in your life right now that you need to resolve or address?
- When and how will you spend time working on these issues?
- How will you switch them off again so that you can focus on your performance?

Re-energising your performance focus

Mentally tough performers are acutely aware of the importance of not only switching their performance focus on, but also switching it off. This may be at the end of each day, or it could be over more prolonged periods such as holidays when restoration is the number one priority. This minimises the risk of burn-out and also reflects a balanced perspective on life, making time for the other things and people that matter outside the performance environment. Work/life balance has been a common topic in my one-to-one coaching with senior executives desperately searching for the 'magic formula' for getting it right. Sadly, many do not achieve the successful balance they are striving for, and this can have dire consequences for their home life and sometimes their performance at work. The following approaches are particularly useful in being able to switch off from the pressure of delivering sustained high performance, and also helping you achieve a healthy work/life balance.

Planning restoration periods. Restoration is crucial in the sustained high performance delivery process. Just as your body needs rest so that it can recharge its energy resources, so does your mind. Relentless pressure will take its toll in the form of mental fatigue and reduced concentration capability. It becomes more difficult to focus over sustained periods and the only answer is a time-out. Relaxing holidays are one obvious means of restoring the mind's energy in readiness for a renewed challenge. Planning regular holidays in your calendar is an important way of re-energising your focus. Another way is to plan 'quiet' times in your weekly schedule where you will not think about work.

Planning enjoyment time. A very pleasant way of re-energising your focus is to plan times when you will simply enjoy yourself. The activities you engage in will be specific to your needs and 'what turns you on', but they provide attractive opportunities to switch off from any performance-related pressure. They also provide an important opportunity to be with people who are important outside the performance environment and to establish what is an appropriate work/life balance. One thing to bear in mind is that enjoyment often involves mental exertion, maybe in the form of competitive sport, playing musical instruments and socialising, so it forms a vehicle for switching focus from one thing to another rather than winding down energy expenditure. As such, it serves as a way of distracting you from the pressure.

Pressing the focus on-off switch. I described earlier in this chapter how using a light switch, either physically or metaphorically, can be a helpful technique for switching your performance focus on. The light switch can also be used to turn your performance focus off, giving you the opportunity to focus on restoration and enjoyment activities. This will prove particularly useful in the early stages of establishing a better work/life balance.

Over to Adrian . . .

All these techniques are ones that I have spent years working on. I think that I have carried over many of them into my working life now – particularly the 'on-off switch'! I use the analogy of the video recorder actually, and put myself on pause every now and then. As I mentioned earlier, I do see this as a particularly important skill. I am at my best when I block out some restoration time. For me, this could be as simple as reading the paper or a novel on a train or plane journey, rather than feeling that I have to look at business papers. I also switch off my phone for the odd half hour!

At a macro level I plan and keep to my holidays. I take every day I am allowed, and again I never take any work papers or even my phone. When we started Lane4 I forgot some of these basic principles, and became quite overloaded and stressed. It wasn't until I managed my time more effectively that I became more productive.

These techniques and strategies relating to restoration and enjoyment time-outs are little more than common sense. However, when under pressure over prolonged periods, you may forget about your need for them and you just haven't got time for them anyway! This is when you most need these time-outs and planning them into your diary might be the only way of ensuring that they happen. The distinction between restoration and enjoyment is important. Restoration involves allowing your mind to wind down and not taxing it too much; it is quite literally about allowing it to rest. Enjoyment time can involve your mind being just as active as when you are in the busiest moments in your performance environment, but it takes your mind off the pressures. These techniques and strategies therefore help you in different ways, and are both valuable and should be built into your life. The light switch metaphor can aid this process in the early stages of getting used to switching into these different modes. Use Time-Out 7.5 to think about ways of managing and planning your time better so that restoration becomes a natural part of your working life.

Time-Out 7.5

Re-energising your performance focus

- How much restoration time have you got planned in the diary at the moment? Do you need to plan some more?
- How much time do you set aside to enjoy yourself and switch off from your job? Do you need to plan some enjoyment time?
- If the light switch metaphor does not work for you in helping to switch your focus on and off, what else might you try?

Not getting derailed by success and failure

Both failure and success bring with them the risk of being a distraction to future performance. Performers can be paralysed by failure or become carried away and excited by success. Mentally tough performers allocate a period of time following important events to deal with their failures and successes. They seldom 'beat themselves up' after failures, but they *are* careful to identify and analyse the causes. This process involves drawing out the learning points before leaving the failures behind as history and moving on armed with their learning.

Mentally tough performers also ensure that they make time to celebrate and enjoy their successes. I have witnessed performers put as much effort into their celebrations as they did into their successful performance! And why not? They work hard to deliver the highest levels of performance and deserve to enjoy their achievements. These performers don't move on without scrutinising and thoroughly understanding the reasons underpinning their success. In this way they are able to build further on their strengths, and recognise and continually replicate those things that are the key to their achievements. This is an important distinguishing factor between performers who are merely 'good' and those who are 'great'; the lesser performers tend to focus on dissecting their failures and may forget about understanding their successes.

The key messages for you in dealing with success and failure so that you can re-focus on the next performance are as follows:

In the case of failure:

- Do not beat yourself up!
- Identify and analyse the causes.

- Draw out the learning points to take forward.
- Leave the failure behind as history.

In the case of success:

- Spend time celebrating it!
- Scrutinise and understand the reasons for your success.
- Use these reasons to build on your strengths and to reproduce in future performances.

Over to Adrian . . .

The hunger to be the best can sometimes drive you forward without 'stopping to appreciate the view'! As you have read, not only is this critical for building future belief, but it is critical to understand how you have been successful and how you can replicate it. We would always review races, or indeed entire 'campaigns' (an Olympics cycle) to see how things could get better. This was possibly taken to the extreme after I won the Olympics in 1988, when after a particularly relaxed bout of parties and celebrations I couldn't stop thinking of how, in the build-up to the race, I had got this part wrong, or that part. I remember sitting in a hotel room a little the worse for wear, thinking that I should really go train with the Australians who had developed a new training method . . .!

These processes will ensure you deal fully with any failure or success so that you don't carry any unwanted disappointment or despondency on the one hand, or perhaps complacency on the other, into the next performance. Work through Time-Out 7.6 to reflect on how you currently deal with success and failure and how you might enhance your strategies in the future.

Time-Out 7.6

Not getting derailed by success and failure

- Think about a recent success:

  Did you spend time scrutinising and understanding the reasons for your success?

  Did you celebrate it?

  How do you want to do things differently following your next success?

- Think about a recent failure:

  Did you beat yourself up?

  Did you identify and analyse the causes?

  Did you draw out the learning points to take forward?

  Did you leave the failure behind as history?

  How do you want to do things differently following your next failure?

Switching focus

You will have gathered by now that focus is a complex area to get to grips with. It gets even more complex when you consider that many situations require performers to be able to switch their focus very rapidly between different elements of the environment that each provide key information required to make decisions, determine the next action and so on. Consider, for example, the demands on a footballer in possession of the ball. He must switch his focus back and forth, and very rapidly, between information from many different sources that include: the ball at his feet; the positions and movements of opponents in close proximity who may attempt to take the ball away from him; the positions and movements of his teammates in relation to opponents so that he can pick out the most appropriate player to pass the ball to; the calls from different teammates who may want him to pass the ball to them, etc.

A number of years ago, American psychologist Robert Nideffer proposed a framework[30] that I have adopted in helping performers simplify and understand this complex phenomenon. It also explains how some performers might find such rapid switches in focus easier than others.

[30] Robert Nideffer, *The Inner Athlete: Mind Plus Muscle For Winning*, Crowell, 1976.

Nideffer identified focus as varying along two continua.

1 'Width', ranging from **broad** (focusing on several things at the same time) to **narrow** (focusing on one or a small number of things at any one time).
2 'Direction', ranging from **internal** (focusing on one's thoughts and feelings) to **external** (focusing on things in the external environment).

Figure 7.2 shows the two continua and how focus can be broken down into four areas or quadrants. The figure also includes the example of the footballer in possession of the ball to demonstrate the essential differences between the areas of focus in the four quadrants.

- The footballer's focus in **quadrant 1** (broad-external) is on the 'big picture' factors in the external environment. He must quickly monitor the positions and movements of his teammates in relation to opponents, as well as being aware of calls from his teammates to pass the ball to them.
- The footballer must narrow his focus in **quadrant 2** (narrow-external) to the player he has selected to pass to and the opponent(s) around him, and also the distance the ball must travel to reach him.
- In **quadrant 3** (narrow-internal) the footballer must focus on making the specific movements to get in position to make the pass to his teammate. He might also be aware that he will have to deliver the pass with his non-preferred foot and there may be some doubt about making the pass successfully. Alternatively, he may be making the pass with his stronger foot and be confident in his ability to make the pass.
- Finally, **quadrant 4** (broad-internal) requires a focus on striking the ball so that it arrives at the player's desired destination. At this point the footballer needs to have a trust in himself to 'let it happen'.

This is a very simplified way of looking at the complex demands on the footballer, but it emphasises the importance of being able to switch focus between the quadrants instantly and almost automatically.

Figure 7.2 Focusing on making the perfect pass.

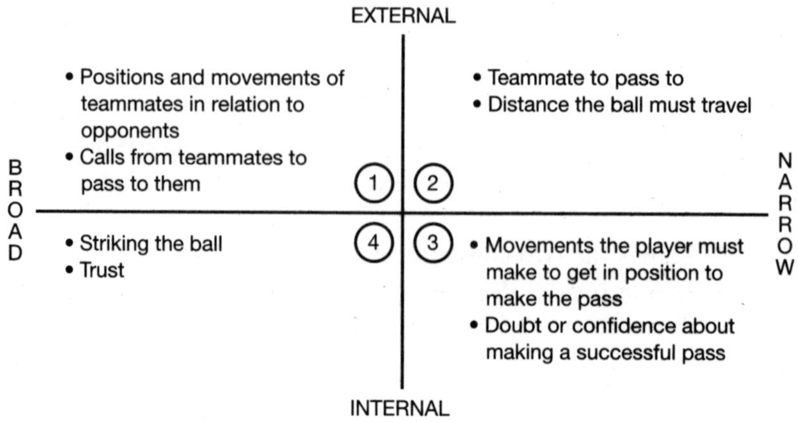

I have worked with performers in the business world who have had similar demands upon them. The framework shown in Figure 7.2 has helped them to structure their focus and be much more aware of the demand to be able to switch it quickly and effectively. For example, equity traders working in particularly volatile markets have to monitor developments in the markets overall (broad-external), and then assess and anticipate the impact they will have on their own equities (narrow-external). In really turbulent times, they may be aware of their own anxiety, perhaps in the form of rapid, shallow breathing or a pounding heart (narrow-internal), but it is important for them to be able to trust themselves and their instinct in the moment (broad-internal).

This focus framework has helped some traders to identify factors they can control, and to better recognise and understand the demands upon them so they can deal more effectively with them under pressure. It has helped some traders recognise tendencies to become 'stuck' in perhaps one or two quadrants, where, for example, they may focus more on their anxiety than on trusting themselves to make the trade.

This framework has also been helpful to executives whose roles do not require quite the same rapid-fire decision-making and action. For example, Barry, a marketing senior executive, found presentations to large audiences quite daunting and tended to spend most of his time focusing on his nerves and general discomfort from actually being in the situation (i.e. quadrant 3: narrow-internal). This reinforces the fact that external factors in the environment are not the only threat to your focus and that an inappropriate inward focus can be equally distracting. Focusing on how nervous you feel or on your doubts can consume your focus to the extent that you may not be able to think about anything else. The major goal that emerged from our coaching sessions was for Barry to focus instead on more positive and facilitative aspects of his thoughts and feelings, as well as making an impact with the audience by being able to also focus on them and their needs.

Figure 7.3 shows the outcome of applying the focus framework to plan for a particularly significant presentation that was looming. We initially worked on identifying more positive thoughts and feelings (quadrant 3 – narrow-internal focus) that would help Barry in delivering his presentation. His new focus would be on feeling prepared, in control and confident; Barry labelled this focus 'how I want to feel inside'. We then worked on being able to focus on other important elements of the presentation. Quadrant 4 (broad-internal), 'how I want to appear', was essentially about his behaviour and actions in the form of being relaxed, approachable, enjoying the experience and 'knowing his stuff'. His focus in quadrant 1 (broad-external), 'focus on big picture', was on the experience of the audience as a whole in terms of his desire for them to enjoy it, to be inspired, to be able to interact with himself and one another and to be able to translate his key messages into action. Barry also wanted to appeal to individuals within the audience and so his focus in quadrant 2 (narrow-external), 'focus in on individuals', was having empathy for the different needs or circumstances of individuals.

Barry worked hard at structuring the content and his rehearsal of the presentation around the different types of focus, ensuring a balance across the four areas. The presentation turned out to be 'the best I have ever delivered' because Barry had learned and grasped the notion of being able to switch focus, and to shake off his tendency to focus in quadrant 3.

Figure 7.3 Focusing on making a great presentation.

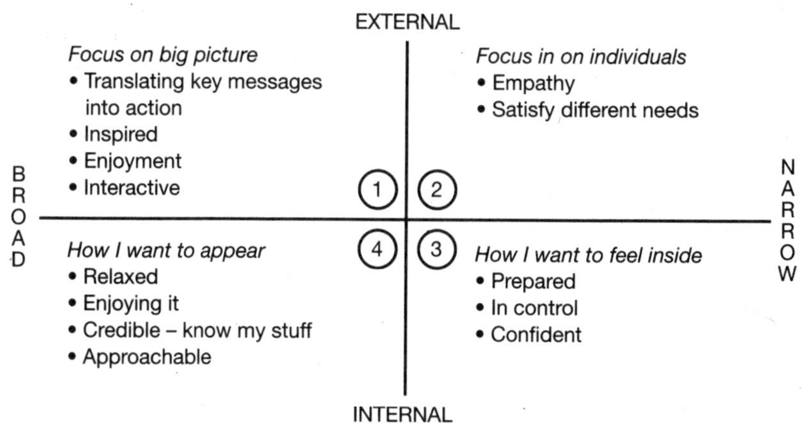

Time-Out 7.7 enables you to apply this framework in assessing where your own focus is when you are successful, and to compare it with times when you are not successful.

Time-Out 7.7

Switching focus

Think about a recent performance that went well and when you were pleased with yourself.

- Where was your focus and what happened to it during the performance?
- Try to compartmentalise your areas of focus at this time in the appropriate quadrants in the framework below.
- Which quadrant(s) did you spend most of your time in, and what was the content of your focus in these different quadrants?

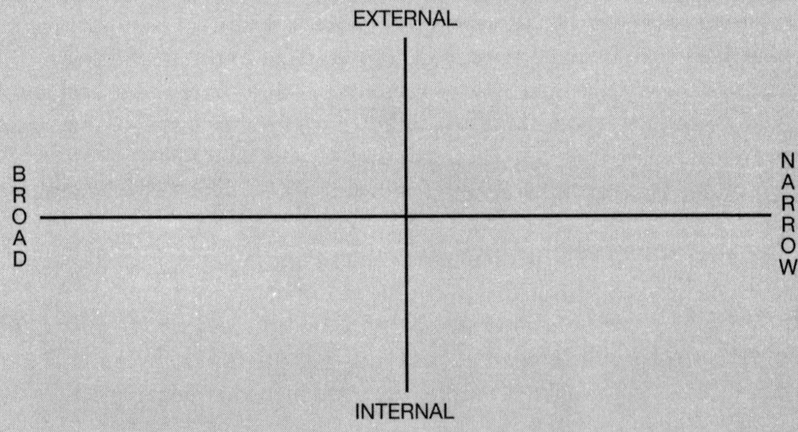

Now think about another time when the same, or similar, performance was not successful.

- Where was your focus then, and what happened to it during the performance?
- Again, try to compartmentalise your areas of focus at this time in the appropriate quadrants in the framework.
- Which quadrant(s) did you spend most of your time in, and what was the content of your focus in these different quadrants?

What were the key differences in your focus in the two performances?

I am confident that your focus will have been different in some way in the two scenarios. Be aware of your focus during the successful performance, and how you achieved it, because this is what you want to reproduce in the future. Think about how you might use some of the techniques and strategies described earlier in this chapter to help you shift between quadrants and, if necessary, to change the content of your focus in those quadrants to achieve optimal performance.

Focusing style

The previous section explored how your focus often needs to switch rapidly during specific situations. Nideffer's original work was based on the premise that people have a *style* of directing their focus. In other words, you may have a tendency, or even a preference, to spend more time in one or two of the quadrants than the others. You may be in a job or role that suits your particular style. For example, if you are an accountant whose style is to focus mainly in the narrow-external quadrant, then this will be a benefit in processing details and numbers accurately. If your style as an accountant was to operate in the broad-external quadrant, then the proposal is that you would struggle to stick with the detail over prolonged periods. The exercise in the previous section may provide some clues as to your focusing style, if you have one.

Over to Adrian . . .

Understanding how to switch my attention and focus during very important moments was one of the biggest lessons I ever learned. It was also one of the hardest. Not only that, but it is easily one of the most transferable skills in dealing with the many sources of input, or information, that I am faced with in my current job. I have to write a proposal, but my phone just rang. Not only that, but I can see someone hovering outside my office. Then I start thinking about that concert I will be meeting my wife at tonight . . . It is endless. Thoughts inside my head, sights and sounds outside my head!

As swimmers, we used Nideffer's grid firstly as a conscious awareness-raising tool; asking ourselves questions as to where we are at various times during performances – and where we should be! Before a race it is useful if we are narrow-internal in the minute before the gun goes off. Then broad-internal in the moment it does! At work now, I find myself in the broad-external quadrant quite a lot, thinking about our strategy and the market conditions and, as a Managing Director, you might expect me to. But the need to switch to a narrow-external focus in the form of something like a more specific customer plan constantly beckons. Recognising where your focus is and being able to switch it around the various quadrants as appropriate was crucial in my swimming successes and it is equally important in my current world.

Chris Andy Scott Emma Studies

Chris

Chris quickly recognised that his focus had been 'pulled' from an internal perspective - being his own man - to listening to and acting on advice that was flooding in from the external environment. He had become interested in what journalists were writing about him in the newspapers; he had been trying to achieve the impossible task of placating a variety of stakeholders who were out for his blood. Chris' realisation that this was merely a distraction from his objective of building a strong foundation for the future success of the team led him to identify those things that really mattered and that he could control. He accepted the criticism as part of the job and used the trigger question 'am I focusing on what really matters?' to re-focus on those things when necessary.

Chris also learned to switch off from his job and give his performance focus a time-out to re-energise. The light switch metaphor worked particularly well in this respect for turning his performance focus both off and then back on again.

Andy

The focus framework described earlier in this chapter (see Figures 7.2 and 7.3) proved to be an excellent vehicle for enabling Andy to control his focus in situations that had caused him problems. In the same way that Barry (described earlier in this chapter) used the framework to enhance his presentation delivery, so Andy employed it to establish how he wanted 'to be' in the presence of his board team. His focus in the narrow-internal area would be on the specific underpinnings of a renewed self-belief and confidence in himself. In the broad-internal area he focused on a general feeling of enjoying being in the role. Inspiring people with his vision for the company was his broad-external focus, while his focus in the narrow-external area was on understanding individual needs of his board members. This approach enabled Andy to go into work each day in a much more positive frame of mind which greatly enhanced his presence and performance.

Scott

For Scott, the game of golf he once loved had sadly become something he dreaded. He had been taking his financial difficulties and worries with him out on to the golf course, and his focus was about winning and nothing else. The first step in becoming more mentally tough in this area was to recognise that this focus was inappropriate and only served to put even more pressure on him. Scott then identified what he wanted to focus on and came up with a list that comprised the following:

- Focus on what I can control - my performance and no one else's!
- Focus on process - smooth, relaxed swing.
- Stay in the moment - what's gone is history, what will happen depends on what I do right now.
- Stay in control - use my breathing technique.

Scott carried this list with him on the course and occasionally glanced at it as a reminder when he was under pressure.

Emma

Emma's focus was on being someone and something she was not. This was initially caused by her intense focus on the external environment and how she thought she was perceived. Having worked out that her perceptions had probably been distorted by her own anxiety about being a woman in a male-dominated environment, Emma turned her focus inward towards just 'being herself' and doing the things that were natural to her and had enabled her success to date. She quickly became much more comfortable in her surroundings and relations with her peers improved dramatically.

In a nutshell

- Focus is about clear and vivid thoughts and images that occupy your conscious mind, and involves withdrawing your thoughts and images from some things to deal effectively with others.
- Focus is a limited capacity resource so where you allocate it is crucial.
- Focusing on the potential of making mistakes increases the probability of making them.
- High achievers, when under pressure, tend to focus on controllables rather than non-controllables, and on processes, the present, positives and staying composed.
- Mental toughness is about
  - being able to shut out distractions;
  - being able to recover from unexpected, uncontrollable events;
  - focusing on your own performance;
  - not letting personal life distractions get in the way;
  - re-energising your performance focus;
  - not getting derailed by success and failure.
- Successful performance often requires you to switch your focus rapidly between broad-internal, broad-external, narrow-internal and narrow-external elements of yourself and the environment.

→ What next?

- Learn to recognise the difference in your focus when you are successful and unsuccessful.
- Experiment with the different techniques and strategies described in this chapter to achieve a focus that will deliver success.
- Don't forget to give your performance focus a rest from time to time.

8 Frequently-Asked Questions About Mental Toughness

After reading this chapter you will know about:

- The importance of being mentally tough but not 'going over the top'
- What to expect as you develop your mental toughness
- Mental toughness in teams

You have now reached the point where you know a lot about mental toughness and its four pillars. This book has guided you through a process of reflecting on just how mentally tough you are and you have hopefully been working on aspects that will enhance your ability to deliver sustained high performance under pressure. You may have decided to work on one or two key elements that will help you deal better with specific circumstances or situations, or you may have decided to work progressively on all of the pillars of mental toughness.

My experience of running workshops on mental toughness is that after working through the four pillars, people have a number of questions about the development of mental toughness and its potential impact. This final chapter addresses the questions I have been most often asked, specifically:

- What difference will it *really* make if I improve my mental toughness?
- Can you be *too* mentally tough?
- Just how easy is it to develop mental toughness?
- What about mental toughness in teams?
- How is mental toughness different from emotional intelligence?

What difference will it *really* make if I improve my mental toughness?

Providing you have the necessary skills and competencies to perform your role, mental toughness is the key to delivering high performance that is sustainable. Just look at what it enables you to do:

- thrive on, rather than merely cope with pressure;
- maintain belief in yourself when it is being seriously challenged;
- achieve a level and type of motivation that works *for* rather than *against* you;
- stay focused on the things that matter in the face of a multitude of potential distractions.

Research carried out by Lane4 provides strong evidence that being mentally tough really does make a difference. Separate studies of sales people operating in a highly competitive market and elite global market traders resulted in self-generated definitions of mental toughness in their roles as:

> *the ability to respond positively to multiple and sometimes conflicting pressures and deliver consistently successful performance*

and

> *the ability to perform at consistently high levels through times of personal and professional pressure*

respectively. The sales force study also showed that people formally classified as 'high performers' in the organisation scored higher on all of the mental toughness pillars than peers who were not classified as 'high performers'. These findings reveal two factors that are particularly important.

1 Mental toughness really is vital in helping people to deal effectively with pressure.

2 Mental toughness is a distinguishing factor between high performers and those who are not delivering the same levels of performance on a consistent basis.

Over to Adrian . . .

One of the reasons I am involved in this book is because I firmly believe that the frameworks and skills outlined in it can be used by anyone, no matter what their performance environment. I also know that developing myself in these ways led directly to my successes, both in the pool and now as a business leader.

More and more organisations are at last beginning to recognise that the high demands they impose on their people are creating pressure that challenges even their very best performers. The importance of mental toughness is reflected in the fact that these organisations are now willing to invest in equipping their people with mental toughness across different market sectors and at all levels in order to meet such challenges effectively and efficiently.

Can you be **too** mentally tough?

I alluded to the danger of associating mental toughness with the extremes of human endeavour in Chapter 3. The essential underpinnings are the same, but 'everyday' mental toughness is not about choosing to place your health, well-being or even life at risk. For people who are mentally tough day-in day-out, common sense almost always prevails.

This question is essentially about the difference between being mentally tough and mentally weak. Confusion occurs when, paradoxically, weakness is misconstrued as strength. Here are some weaknesses that might be inappropriately associated with mental toughness.

- Being so focused on your performance that you ignore everything else going on in your life or what is happening around you.
- Being so entrenched in your own view of the world that you will not budge from it.
- Having a self-belief that is based solely on tangible achievements and can only be fed by further material gains.
- Being under stress and denying it.
- Having an intense motivation or desire that is fuelled by fear of failure and perhaps avoidance.

- Continuing to push yourself hard when it is clear to everyone else that it is futile and can only endanger your health or well-being.
- Making sacrifices rather than choices.

In other words, I do not believe that you can be too mentally tough as such. The danger is in misconstruing mental toughness as those attributes and other similar ones above. They merely constitute mental weakness!

Over to Adrian . . .

I referred earlier in the book to times when I was too focused on success, and the negative impact it had – not only on myself, but those around me. In losing my first Olympics I had also overlooked key stages of overtraining, because I wanted to appear to be 'tough', but the tougher thing would have been to rest!

Just how easy is it to develop mental toughness?

Developing mental toughness is not necessarily easy, otherwise everyone would be mentally tough and you would not be reading this! This book has described how you can become more mentally tough following a structured approach to enhancing each of the four pillars. This process does not always involve continual forward progress. None of the people described in the **C**hris **A**ndy **S**cott **E**mma Studies in the earlier chapters found their development straightforward and easy. For a couple of them, they may actually have taken a step backwards before they made any significant progress. The process sometimes involved delving deep within to raise their awareness and understanding of what was happening to them and how they needed to change their thoughts, attitudes and behaviours. This sometimes caused confusion as they sought answers that were not obvious. They progressed through a series of stages, shown in Figure 8.1, that first of all involved **acceptance** of the need to become mentally tough. They then entered the stage of **exploration**, in which they experimented with different strategies and techniques. Gradually, they found things that worked for them and entered the stage of **commitment** in which they practised and honed those strategies and techniques that worked in different situations, with different people, and so on. Finally, they reached the stage of **continuous growth**, by which time they had enhanced their mental toughness, and were using techniques and strategies that were finely tuned and directed at even further development.

Over to Adrian . . .

It *is* hard, but it's also achievable. For me, it is an ongoing process too, honing and building on things I already know. I worked on the psychology of performance as a swimmer for over ten years. Again, it's not easy, but nothing worthwhile ever is! I would absolutely recommend that you start the journey though.

An important aspect of **C**hris, **A**ndy, **S**cott and **E**mma's development was to take small steps and to build gradually on these. A couple of them found documenting their experiences and associated learnings particularly helpful in monitoring and demonstrating their progress.

Figure 8.1 The key steps to developing mental toughness.

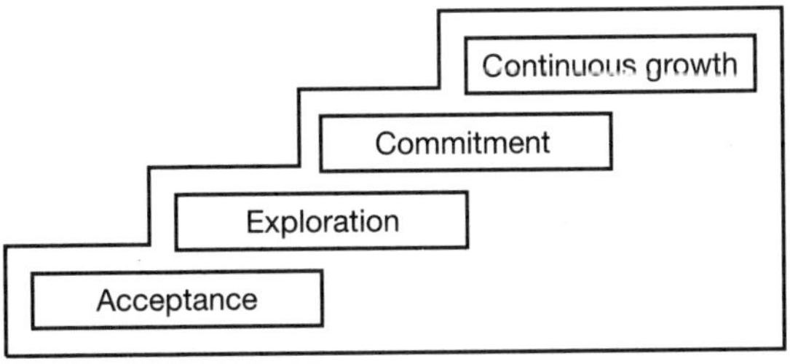

What about mental toughness in teams?

The focus of this book has been on developing mental toughness at an individual level. However, I am frequently asked if there is such a thing as a 'mentally tough team'. Although there is no useful research evidence around to provide a definitive answer, I firmly believe that mentally tough teams *do* exist and that they are underpinned by the same four pillars that underpin mental toughness in individuals.

Firstly, mentally tough teams have a strong collective belief in a number of areas, including their ability to deliver high performance on a sustained basis, belief in one another's capability and belief in the designated leader. This collective belief is backed up by robust self-belief in individual team members that enables them to both offer and ask for advice, support and coaching from others in the team. This belief sustains their commitment, determination and focus when times are hard. It also enables openness and challenge that form the foundation of the team's further growth.

Secondly, the motivation of all team members is reflected in a strong commitment to collective goals and needs that are actually prioritised above their own. However, mentally tough teams also work hard at aligning team and individual aspirations so that they complement one another rather than cause conflict. Indeed, such teams work hard to support one another in striving to hit individual targets so that all team members' achievements result in a shared sense of pride and success. Mentally tough teams learn from setbacks and use it as the basis of an enhanced determination to succeed in the future. They also deal well with challenge and even conflict, recognising that it can serve an important purpose and help in the team's further growth.

Thirdly, mentally tough teams are highly resilient and supportive of one another when under pressure. There is a heavy emphasis on caring for team members' well-being with support being constantly available for individuals or units who find themselves in difficult situations. These teams are good at helping one another with the symptoms of pressure, and sometimes stress, but are always keen to tackle the sources of pressure. Pressure is openly talked about and monitored so that action can be taken when required.

Finally, mentally tough teams are not easily distracted from their purpose. They focus on controllables rather than wasting valuable energy on things they have no influence over. They focus on maximising supports and minimising constraints. They 'share' their focus around team members so that they have all the angles covered. In this way all members assume an accountability and responsibility that ensures the team remains on course towards achieving its goals. Mentally tough teams also have carefully considered and prepared responses for dealing with different circumstances that may arise so that they are not easily derailed when things do not go as planned.

Over to Adrian . . .

Contrary to popular belief, I have always believed swimming to be a team sport! Even though I would mostly race individually (with the odd relay), I spent most of my waking life in training or travelling to competitions in a team. In my time in the City of Leeds team over a five year period, we were consistently in the top three in the European club championships. In the year we won, I know that we exhibited a collective sense of belief and shared pressures equally.

How is mental toughness different from emotional intelligence?

People who are familiar with emotional intelligence sometimes challenge me about how mental toughness is different. There are some common elements, but there are fundamental differences that mean that they should be treated as two separate disciplines. The notion of emotional intelligence was originally developed in the 1970s and 80s but was not brought to the attention of a non-academic audience until the publication of Daniel Goleman's book, *Emotional Intelligence*, in 1995. Since then emotional intelligence has been the subject of several refinements and modifications by others who have also realised its potential to help business executives to function better in organisational contexts.

Emotional intelligence is based on the premise that academic intelligence, otherwise known as IQ, does not necessarily predict success in a business context. Proponents argue, instead, that emotional intelligence is the better predictor since it includes essential awareness and behavioural elements that enhance understanding of yourself and others. Goleman articulated five domains of emotional intelligence as:

- knowing your emotions;
- managing your emotions;
- motivating yourself;
- recognising and understanding other people's emotions;
- managing relationships.

As such, emotional intelligence is about understanding and managing yourself and relationships with others.

Over to Adrian . . .

Like Graham, I think that emotional intelligence and mental toughness are different, but I also believe that I would not have achieved the same level of success if I didn't have strength in both. In common is the self-awareness piece, and for me it is the starting point to any great performer's progression towards success. But it is not sufficient, on its own, to deliver sustained high performance under pressure. That's where mental toughness comes to the fore.

Mental toughness *does* involve an enormous element of self-awareness, like emotional intelligence, but the focus is much more on self-management than management of others. The fundamental differences between them are twofold. Firstly, mental toughness is about how you respond to and deal with pressure and the accompanying environment. Secondly, mental toughness is about performance – delivering high performance that is sustainable. In this way, mental toughness is much more than just being emotionally intelligent.

A final word from Adrian . . .

The most important thing about mental toughness is that it becomes a part of you rather than a thing that you just switch on. It is also worth remembering that it is a complex area and it is not something that you can learn overnight. In essence it is the ability to reflect on your experiences and draw sense from them using a simple framework. Not only are self-belief, motivation, handling pressure and being focused important in their own right, but there is an interaction between them. I am more likely to handle pressure when I walk into a situation believing in myself, and being able to focus on the moment in front of me, than just thinking in a linear way.

I also strongly believe that it is possible to develop mental toughness. But as with any development, you have to start with a good level of self-awareness and humility to recognise you have to do something different. In my situation I learnt most things from failures, and being upfront in analysing them and taking responsibility for making a change.

As a swimmer I believed that my 'mental training' was equally as important as my swimming or 'physical' training. If I only did the yards in the pool, I would have been half a competitor. It's the same in business now. As an MD I can gain skills and experience, and as a consultant I can develop ways of working with clients, but if I haven't developed and spent time working on those key aspects of mental toughness, then I know I will be less impactful. Work just wouldn't be as much fun either.

In a nutshell

- Mental toughness *really does* make a difference. Research has shown that it distinguishes between high performers and those who are not delivering the same levels of performance on a consistent basis.
- It is important to identify signs of mental weakness and not confuse them with mental toughness.
- Mental toughness is not necessarily easy to develop, but it *is* worth the effort!
- Mental toughness can exist at a team level.
- Mental toughness is much more than just being emotionally intelligent.

Wrap-up

If there is one thing that will really take you to another level of performance – to the plateau where your victories are measured in the blink of milliseconds – it might be the ability to embrace pressure, to understand it, to draw it in, to make it your own, and use it to your advantage...We've been trained to think of pressure as the enemy, the unfair burden that holds us down...Pressure is nothing more than the shadow of great opportunity.

Michael Johnson[31]

Good luck and be mentally tough.

[31] Michael Johnson, *Slaying the Dragon*, Harper Collins, 1996, pp. 179–180.

Appendix A: Meditative Relaxation

Background

Meditation has been around in one form or another for at least 5,000 years. It has traditionally been associated with spiritual purposes, but its recent widespread use outside of any religious framework reflects the large number of people who use meditation as part of a personal growth process or, quite simply, to relax. Meditation was popularised a number of years ago as Transcendental Meditation, or TM, in which you repeat silently to yourself and focus on a mantra word. Research[32] has shown that TM used with the mantra 'one' on each exhalation has the following benefits:

- reduced heart rate;
- reduced blood pressure;
- lower oxygen consumption;
- decreased metabolic rate;
- reduced concentration of lactic acid in the blood (associated with lower anxiety);
- increased electrical resistance in the skin (associated with deep relaxation);
- increased alpha wave activity in the brain (associated with relaxed states);
- increased energy levels;
- heightened alertness;
- reduced self-criticism;
- increased objectivity (i.e. viewing situations non-judgmentally);

---

[32] Herbert Benson, *Beyond the Relaxation Response*, Morrow, 1975.

- heightened self-esteem;
- increased accessibility of emotions.

Guidelines for practising meditation[33]

- Find a quiet environment where you will not be disturbed.
- Try not to meditate on a full stomach.
- Ideally, you should wear loose clothing, but if this is not feasible, then at least remove your shoes and loosen your belt if you notice any tightness around your waist.
- Find yourself a comfortable position. You will find it easier to meditate in the early stages if you lie on a sofa or bed. Do not cross your feet, arms or legs.
- It may help if you place your hands on your stomach to enable you to feel the steady rhythm of your breaths in and out.
- You may experience feeling heavy or perhaps a light, floating sensation. These are normal experiences. If you experience anything that is remotely unpleasant, then stop meditating.
- If you are distracted by any noises or thoughts, don't try to ignore them. Instead, let them pass and gently bring your intended focus back again.
- Approach it with a non-judgmental, passive attitude. If you think it won't work, then it won't work!
- Try to meditate every day. You will get better as you practise it.
- Meditation is often easier if you keep your eyes closed during it.

Deep relaxation

Set aside at least 15 minutes for the session. It will be helpful in the early stages if you record an audio tape to guide you through the meditation process. Follow the process below.

---

[33] Meditation can release emotions that cause problems for people with a history of mental illness. In these circumstances, medical advice should be sought before practising meditative relaxation.

Make yourself comfortable.

(30 second interval)

Close your eyes and focus on your breathing.

(Continue for 1 minute)

Now focus on saying 'one' to yourself as you breathe out.

(Continue for 5 minutes)

Now focus on counting down from ten to one on successive breaths out until you reach one and continue with one.

(When you reach one continue for five minutes)

Now focus on counting up from one to seven on successive breaths in. Take deeper breaths as you count up.

On seven open your eyes.

Intermediate relaxation

Set aside at least five minutes for the session. It will be helpful in the early stages if you record an audio tape to guide you through the meditation process. Follow the process below.

Make yourself comfortable.

(30 second interval)

Close your eyes and focus on your breathing.

(Continue for 30 seconds)

Now focus on saying 'one' to yourself as you breathe out.

(Continue for one minute)

Now focus on counting down from five to one on successive breaths out until you reach one and continue with one.

(When you reach one continue for two minutes)

Now focus on counting up from one to three on successive breaths in. Take deeper breaths as you count up.

On three open your eyes.

Quick relaxation

This form of relaxation can be practised in most situations and circumstances, but obviously not when you might put yourself in danger (e.g. when driving a car). Follow the process below.

Close your eyes or focus on a small object that is static.
Focus on saying 'one' to yourself on each breath out.
Continue for three or four breaths.
Open your eyes or stop focusing on the small object.

Appendix B: Imagery-Based Relaxation

Imagery-based relaxation involves focusing on a relaxing image. The image might be a quiet beach, beautiful countryside, mountains, your bedroom, a cozy fire, etc. The image doesn't have to reflect reality. Floating on a cloud or flying on a magic carpet can be just as powerful in inducing a relaxed state – it's your choice. The key is to visualise the scene in as much detail as possible so that you become absorbed in it. This will reduce any physical tension you are experiencing. You might want to record a script of the relaxing scene on an audio tape and then use it to guide you through it. An example of a relaxing scene is provided below.

> *You're strolling along a beautiful deserted beach. You are barefoot and can feel the soft white sand beneath your feet as you walk along the water's edge. You can hear the sound of the surf as the waves ebb and flow. The sound is hypnotic, relaxing you more and more. The water is a beautiful greeny-blue flecked with white caps far out where the waves are cresting. The sound of the waves breaking on the shore lulls you deeper and deeper into relaxation. You draw in the fresh, salty smell of the air with each breath. Your skin glows with the warmth of the sun. You can feel a gentle breeze against your cheek and ruffling your hair. Take in the whole scene as you feel very calm and at ease.*

An important point about the above script is that it uses language and words that appeal to the senses of sight, touch, hearing and smell. Multisensory words increase the power of the image so that you can experience it as if you were actually there, thus making it conducive to relaxation.

Try designing your own image. Describe it in vivid detail and make sure that it appeals to as many different senses as possible. What does it look like? Are there any sounds? What is the temperature? What are you in physical contact with? What does the air smell like? What colours are prominent?

Appendix C: Progressive Muscular Relaxation (PMR)

Background

PMR involves tensing and relaxing different muscle groups in the body and working through the body in a progressive fashion. It is a particularly effective technique for people whose anxiety is strongly associated with muscle tension or the feelings of being 'uptight' or 'tense'. Tightness in the shoulders and neck, backaches, muscle spasms and insomnia are amongst the symptoms that can be alleviated by employing PMR. Long-term benefits[34] of practising PMR include:

- reduced anxiety;
- reduced panic attacks;
- improved concentration;
- increased control over moods;
- increased self-esteem.

Guidelines for practising PMR

- Find a quiet environment where you will not be disturbed.
- Practise PMR on an empty stomach.
- Ideally, you should wear loose clothing, but if this is not feasible then at least remove your shoes and loosen your belt if you notice any tightness around your waist.

[34] Edmund Jacobson, *Progressive Relaxation*, University of Chicago Press, 1974.

- Find yourself a comfortable position on a rug. Do not cross your feet, arms or legs.
- Approach it with a non-judgmental, passive attitude. If you think it won't work, then it won't work!
- Try to practise PMR every day. You will get better as you practise it.
- When you tense a particular muscle group, do so vigorously, but without straining, for 7–10 seconds.
- Release the tension in the muscle groups immediately and then relax for at least 15-20 seconds before progressing to the next muscle group.
- Allow the muscle groups not being tensed to remain as relaxed as possible.

Deep relaxation

Set aside at least 15 minutes for the session. It will be helpful in the early stages if you record an audio tape to guide you through the PMR process. Follow the process below.

Take three deep abdominal breaths, exhaling slowly each time. Imagine the tension in your body flowing away with each breath out.

Clench your fist. Hold for seven to ten seconds and then release for 15–20 seconds (use the same time periods for the remaining muscle groups).

Tighten your biceps by drawing your forearms up towards your shoulders and 'making a muscle'. Hold...and then relax.

Tighten your triceps – the muscles on the undersides of your upper arms – by extending your arms out straight and locking your elbows. Hold...and then relax.

Tense the muscles in your forehead by raising your eyebrows as far as you can. Hold...and then relax. Imagine your forehead muscles becoming smooth and relaxed.

Tense the muscles around your eyes by clenching your eyelids tightly shut. Hold...and then relax. Imagine sensations of deep relaxation spreading all around the area of your eyes.

Tighten your jaw by opening your mouth widely so you stretch the hinges of your jaw. Hold…and then relax. Let your lips part and allow your jaw to hang loose.

Tighten the muscles in your back by pulling your head back, as if you were going to touch your head to your back. Focus on tensing the muscles in your neck. Hold…and then relax.

Take a few deep breaths and focus on the weight of your head sinking into the floor.

Tighten your shoulders by raising them up as if you were going to touch your ears. Hold…and then relax.

Tighten the muscles around your shoulder blades by pushing your shoulder blades back as if you were going to touch them together. Hold…and then relax.

Tighten the muscles of your chest by taking in a deep breath. Hold for up to ten seconds and then release slowly. Imagine any excess tension in your chest flowing away with the exhalation.

Tighten your stomach muscles by sucking your stomach in. Hold…and then release. Imagine a wave of relaxation spreading through your abdomen.

Tighten your lower back by arching it up. Hold…and then relax.

Tighten your buttocks by pulling them together. Hold…and then relax.

Squeeze the muscles in your thighs all the way down to your knees. Hold…and then relax.

Tighten your calf muscles by pulling your toes towards you. Hold…and then relax.

Tighten your feet by curling your toes downwards. Hold…and then relax.

Scan your body for any remaining tension and tense and relax any muscle groups where there is still some tension.

Imagine a wave of relaxation spreading through your body, starting at your head and going all the way down to your toes.

Quick relaxation

Quick physical relaxation can be induced in a very short period of time by simply scanning the body for any tension. Tense any muscle group(s) where you are aware of tension. Hold and relax in the same way as described above. You may benefit from doing this twice with the same muscle group.

Appendix D: Abdominal Breathing

Your breathing reflects the level of tension you carry in your body. When you are tense, your breathing usually becomes shallow and rapid, involving the upper chest area only. When you are relaxed, you breathe more fully and deeply, and from your abdomen. The exercise below shows you how to reduce tension by breathing from the abdomen.

Place one hand on your abdomen just below your rib cage.

Inhale slowly and deeply through your nose into the bottom of your lungs. Your hand should actually rise and your chest should move only slightly while your abdomen expands.

When you have taken in a full breath, pause for a moment and then exhale slowly through your nose or mouth. As you exhale, allow your whole body to just 'let go'.

Do ten slow, full abdominal breaths. Keep your breathing smooth and regular. It will help if you count to four on the inhalation and then count to four again on the exhalation. Remember to pause at the end of each inhalation before breathing out.

Practise the breathing exercise for five minutes every day for a couple of weeks. You will improve as you practise and find that it is very beneficial in helping you to reduce any physical tension you experience when under stress.

Index